HEMATOLOGY
AND
IMMUNOLOGY
CONCEPTS FOR NURSING

Joyce P. Griffin, R.N., Ph.D. (C.), C.C.R.N.

Doctoral Candidate in Nursing
New York University
New York, New York

APPLETON-CENTURY-CROFTS/Norwalk, Connecticut

0-8385-3686-7

90 / 10 9 8 7 6 5 4 3 2

Prentice-Hall of Australia, Pty. Ltd., Sydney
Prentice-Hall Canada, Inc.
Prentice-Hall Hispanoamericana, S.A., Mexico
Prentice-Hall of India Private Limited, New Delhi
Prentice-Hall International (UK) Limited, London
Prentice-Hall of Japan, Inc., Tokyo
Prentice-Hall of Southeast Asia (Pte.) Ltd., Singapore
Whitehall Books Ltd., Wellington, New Zealand
Editora Prentice-Hall do Brasil Ltda., Rio de Janeiro

PRINTED IN THE UNITED STATES OF AMERICA

Library of Congress Cataloging-in-Publication Data
Griffin, Joyce P.
  Hematology and immunology.

  Bibliography: p.
  Includes index.
    1. Blood—Diseases—Nursing.   2. Immunologic
diseases—Nursing.   3. Hematology.   4. Immunology.
I. Title.   [DNLM: 1. Hematologic Diseases—nursing.
2. Immunologic Diseases—nursing.   3. Nursing Process.
WY 152.5.G851h]
RC633.G75   1986   616.1'5   86-1053
ISBN 0-8385-3686-7

Design: Jean Sabato-Morley
Cover: Paul Agule

PRINTED IN THE UNITED STATES OF AMERICA

To my family, for their unending support.

Contents

Foreword

The publication of *Hematology and Immunology: Concepts for Nursing* is an important event. The author uses nursing diagnoses to present the medical situation and the nursing needs of clients with hematological and immunological diagnoses. The focus on the book is on the total client and the complex physical and psychological needs these clients offer. The nursing care plan which accompanies selected chapters illustrates very clearly the content of the chapter and shows the nurse how to use the theoretical material presented.

Perhaps one of the strongest points of the book is that the clients live as real people. The human suffering involved in hematological and immunological diseases is intense. Clients may not have heard of the disease before they are diagnosed. Many of the diseases were unknown to medical practice until recently and the interaction of genetic and environmental factors in the etiology and onset of the disease is often unknown. At diagnosis, clients are suddenly confronted with a frightening sounding word, such as lupus, which may have important ramifications not only for their own health, but for that of their children. The author is very sensitive to the suffering and fright that accompany one of these diagnoses and offers positive suggestions to minimize the suffering.

The book presents a vast amount of information on the pathophysiology of the diseases. The information is accurate and presented in a scholarly and readable manner. It was the author's intention to write a volume for the practicing nurse in a tertiary care setting that would enhance practice and the quality of care delivered to this unique group of clients. The book accomplishes these purposes admirably.

The focus on nursing intervention is a tremendous strength of the book. Because the client is so clearly and humanly described, the nursing interventions recommended take on a liveliness that is not commonly found in texts. The reader can picture the clients as real people and can mentally rehearse the interventions that are recommended. This kind of role playing should assure that the interventions enter the nurse's practice more quickly than if the nurse had to memorize them and recall them at the client's bedside.

Patricia Winstead-Fry, R.N., Ph.D.
Chair, Department of Nursing
New York University
New York, New York

Preface

Hematology and immunology is an area of science with great potential as a source of ideas for clinical research. The care of clients with disorders of blood cells and immunodeficiencies, to cite just two examples, is extremely complex. The data base underlying our nursing care is limited, and these gaps in our knowledge offer virtually unlimited possibilities for research. What makes hematology and immunology so exciting is that nursing care can make such a tremendous difference in the level of wellness of these clients. This book is arranged around nursing diagnoses—a relatively new phenomenon in nursing which has contributed so immensely to the validation of our professional uniqueness. Nursing diagnosis is an essential step in the nursing process. Because of the relatively recent birth of nursing diagnoses, there are many clinical problems not yet addressed in the established list. As practitioners, we have an obligation to help in the growth of nursing diagnoses by considering new diagnostic possibilities. These untested diagnoses can then be submitted to the National Clearinghouse for Nursing Diagnosis for testing and eventual acceptance into the established list. I have introduced new diagnoses into this book, as well as established ones and hope that readers will be creative in identifying new nursing diagnoses in the area of hematological and immunological nursing. We need to expand the current data base, to discover new and alternative nursing interventions and the diagnoses will follow.

There have been many people who have made this effort possible. My professional colleagues, especially Susan Ruppert and Barbara Kupferschmid, have offered a constant supply of ideas, encouragement, and humor. Many individuals come to mind who have developed, supported, and served as mentors for my research interests. These highly committed individuals are Drs. Pat Winstead-Fry, Chris Tanner, Joy Calkin, Ada Lindsay, and Pam Mitchell. Two of my friends, B. J. McDonald and Joanne Dunleavey, and my family have provided much support. My editors, initially Rick Weimer and subsequently Stu Horton and Susan Prottas, and their staffs have been most facilitative in making this idea a reality.

Lastly, I offer a note of caution to readers. Nursing is an ever-changing science and the area of hematology and immunology is rapidly evolving. This book is intended to be a guide to the care of the client with heme/immune disease. It is *not* an oncology nursing textbook, and other sources should be consulted for complete information on neoplastic disease, chemotherapy, and care of the cancer client. However, many areas are covered that are pertinent to the oncology nurse's practice, including care of the immunosuppressed and bleeding client, care of the bone marrow transplant client, and transfusion therapy. As nursing becomes more complex and specialized, however, nurses in all areas of practice need to have a data base for care of the client with heme/immune disease.

In the text, the use of the term "client" in place of the term "patient" to identify the health care consumer suggests an autonomous person who has freedom of choice in seeking and selecting assistance. The client is no longer a passive recipient of services but an active participant who assumes responsibility for his choices and also for the consequences of those choices.

For no other reason than to avoid awkward and redundant reading, "she" has been used when referring to the nurse, and "he" when referring to the client. It is hoped that this archaic use of genders does not undermine the effectiveness of this book.

Joyce P. Griffin, R.N., Ph.D. (C.), C.C.R.N.

CHAPTER 1

Hematology and Immunology—The Nursing Process

INTRODUCTION

The incidence of hematological and immunological disorders in hospitals has been increasing steadily over the last few years. The treatment for hematological malignancies, immunodeficiency diseases, and coagulopathies has become more sophisticated, complex, but simultaneously, fraught with complications.

Clients who, as recently as 5 years ago, would have succumbed to their diseases are now surviving as our knowledge base grows. As a result, nurses are becoming increasingly cognizant of hematological/immunological physiology and pathophysiology. As the data base rapidly expands in this area of science, nurses are striving to incorporate this knowledge into their practice. The hematological and immunological systems directly affect all other body functions, a concept that becomes strikingly clear with any disorder of these two systems. This ability to evoke far reaching and systemic manifestations of illness has only recently been discovered as new diseases, such as acquired immune deficiency syndrome (AIDS), comes to the forefront.

Additionally, hematological and immunological disorders are frequent complications of other long-term or life-threatening diseases. A classic example of this is the high incidence of disseminated intravascular coagulation in association with septic shock and adult respiratory distress syndrome.

Nursing care of the client with disorders of the hematological and immunological systems is extremely complex. This book attempts to demystify it by discussing physiology, pathophysiology, specific disorders, and nursing care.

THE NURSING PROCESS

The nursing process describes a method of setting the practice of nursing into motion. Through its five steps—assessment, nursing diagnosis, planning, intervention, and evaluation—the nurse uses systematic observational and problem-solving techniques to identify potential problems and appropriate interventions and to evaluate the effectiveness of these interventions.

Assessment

Assessment is the first phase of the nursing process, and is the deliberate and systematic collection of data to determine a client's current health status, to assess for the presence of stressors, and to evaluate his present and past coping patterns. Data are obtained through four methods: interview, physical examination, observation and review of records.

Interview

A history involves the collection of a predetermined set of facts during the initial contact with a client. Have the client describe the presenting health problem or chief complaint in terms of the following symptom profile:

- date and time of onset of symptoms.
- type of onset: gradual or abrupt.
- course of the problems: continuous or intermittent.
- duration: length of time of each episode; frequency of episodes.
- character: description of quality and severity of symptom.
- interference with usual activities.
- location and relocation patterns.
- associated symptoms.
- precipitating conditions.
- relieving factors.
- obtain information about allergies, current medications. (prescribed and over the counter), past medical history, and family history.

Determine the client's perception of his own health status. Identify stressors as perceived by the client. Direct questions related to:

- perception of major problem or stress area.
- how do the present circumstances differ from the usual pattern of living (life-style patterns).
- past coping patterns—has he ever experienced a similar problem and how did he handle it.
- client expectations—what does he anticipate for himself in the future as a consequence of his present situation.
- motivation—what can he do to help himself.
- what does he expect care givers, family, and friends to do.

The care giver should note the perceptions of stressors for the client by answering the above questions also. Note any discrepancies or distortions between the client's perception and that of the nurse regarding the situation.

Determine other factors that are affecting the individual:

- intrapersonal factors—physical, i.e., range of body function or psychosociocultural, i.e., attitudes and values.
- developmental, i.e., age, degree of normalcy.
- interpersonal—resources and relationship of family, friends, or care givers.
- extrapersonal—resources and relationship of community facilities, finances, employment, or other areas.

Physical Examination*

Skin
Assess the skin for color variations, lesions, scarring, wounds, hair distribution, cellulitis, or ulcers. Note skin turgor.

Ears, Eyes, Nose, and Throat
Assess the client's visual and hearing acuity. Observe for signs of inflammation, icterus, swelling, or nodules. Determine if the client has petechiae, lesions, or areas of tenderness.

Respiratory
Observe the client's pattern of respirations. Is he experiencing orthopnea, dyspnea, or tachypnea? Is he using his accessory muscles? Note expansion of the chest: is it symmetrical? Palpate for transmission of vocal fremitus and diaphragmatic excursion. Auscultate for adventitious breath sounds.

Cardiovascular
Observe for placement of the point of maximal impulse (PMI). Note the presence of heaves, distended neck veins, edema, or signs of phlebitis. Auscultate for murmurs, gallops, pericardial friction rubs, pulses paradoxus, irregular rhythms, and abnormalities in blood pressure.

Gastrointestinal
Assess for the presence of abdominal distention, masses, ascites, peristaltic waves, tenderness, or organ enlargement. Auscultate for bowel sounds. Note the presence of perianal ulcerations from such organisms as *Escherichia coli* or fungi. Does the client have diarrhea or cramps?

Genitourinary
Note the presence of lesions, signs of inflammation, swelling, tenderness, or incontinence.

---

*Discussion of all body systems except for physical examination of the hematological/immunological systems are discussed in a cursory manner as this information is well described in many other texts.

Central Nervous System

Assess cranial nerve function and pupillary reactions. Note any changes in mental status. Evaluate motor function and reflexes.

Hematopoietic/Immunological Systems

Subjective. Has the client noted swelling of glands or excessive bruising or bleeding? Was the bleeding spontaneous or trauma induced? Ask the client if he is suffering from excessive fatigue, dyspnea on exertion, palpitations, frequent infections, fever, weight loss, or diarrhea.

Objective. Inspect and palpate all lymph nodes. Isolated lymph nodes less than 1 cm in size are not usually significant in the adult but may indicate an inflammatory response in the client with cancer. The enlargement of lymph nodes in metastatic cancer is characterized by discrete, nontender, firm or hard nodes with an irregular shape; unilateral, regional nodes will be involved. Inspect for pallor, petechiae, and bleeding.

Acute infections are common in the course of treatment for hematological/immunological diseases. The usual parameters of infection may not be present in clients with decreased granulocytes because of the depressed inflammatory response. Erythema and purulent drainage may not be present. Fever of more than 101 °F is the best indicator that an infection is present. The nurse must perform a scrupulous physical examination, being especially attentive to subtle signs of inflammation. The physical examination may need to be repeated frequently especially when an initial source of the infection is not discernible. Because the client's endogenous microbical flora accounts for 86 percent of the infecting organisms, surveillance cultures (nose, throat, urine, and stool) should be considered along with at least two blood cultures. If an intravenous needle or catheter is in place when the client first becomes febrile, it must be considered as a potential focus of infection which should be removed and cultured.

Closely assess the client for signs of infection with herpes zoster, *Staphylococcus*, *Candida*, and other fungi, all of which are commonly found in immunosuppressed clients. If the client complains of diarrhea and cramps, he may have viral enteritis.

Assess for signs of bleeding that may be in the form of petechiae, purpura, and confluent ecchymoses. A client with a coagulopathy may ooze or hemorrhage from obvious or covert sites—nasogastric tubes, endotracheal tubes, central lines, peripheral intravenous sites, or Foley catheters.

Laboratory Examinations

Hematological System

A *CBC* is a complete blood count and differential count. It includes the following studies: (Table 1–1)

TABLE 1-1. LABORATORY EXAMINATIONS

	Hematological System	
Test	*Normal Range*	*Comments*
RBC count	♂ 4.7–6.1 million/cu mm ♀ 4.2–5.4 million/cu mm	↓ with Anemia, hemorrhage ↑ with Chronic anoxia
Hemoglobin (Hgb)	♂ 14–18 g/dl ♀ 12–16	Same as above
Hematocrit (Hct)	♂ 42–52% ♀ 37–47%	Same as above
Mean corpuscular volume (MCV)	80–95 cu/u	↑ RBC macrocytic ↓ RBC microcytic
Mean corpuscular hemoglobin (MCH)	27–31 pg	
Mean corpuscular hemoglobin concentration (MCHC)	32–36 g/dl (32–36%)	↓ Hypochromic cell
White blood cell count (WBC)	5000–10,000/cu mm	↑ Infection ↓ Bone marrow failure
Reticulocyte counts	0.5–2% of total RBC	↓ Inadequate RBC production ↑ Polycythemia vera
Iron (Fe)	60–190 μg/dl	↓ Iron deficiency anemia
Total iron binding capacity (TIBC)	250–420 μg/dl	Same as above
Serum haptoglobin	100–150 mg	↓ Hemolysis liver disease ↑ Inflammatory diseases
Hemoglobin electrophoresis	Hgb A₁ 95–98% Hgb A₂ 2–3% Hgb F 0.8–2% Hgb S 0% Hgb C 0%	Variations indicate hemoglobinopathies
Direct Coombs' Indirect Coombs'	Negative Negative	To detect antibodies against RBC

	Coagulation Tests	
Test	*Normal Range*	*Comments*
Prothrombin test (PT)	11–12.5 seconds (85–100%)	↑ Deficiency of factors V and VII
Prothrombin time test (PTT)	30–40 seconds	↑ Deficiency of factors II, V, VIII, IX, XI, XII
Platelet count	150,000–400,000/cu mm	↓ Bone marrow failure, hypersplenism, accelerated consumption ↑ Hemorrhage, polycythemia vera, malignancies
Bleeding time	1–9 minutes	↑ Thrombocytopenia, marrow infiltration, inadequate platelet function *(continued)*

TABLE 1-1. (Cont.)

Coagulation Tests		
Test	*Normal Range*	*Comments*
Euglobin lysis time	90 minutes–6 hours	↓ Fibrinolysis
Fibrin degradation products test (FDP)	< 10 μg/ml	↑ DIC, fibrinolysis

Immunological System	

A. Nonspecific immune response tests
  1. Tests of inflammatory response
    WBC count and differential
    C-reactive protein
    complement activity
    erythrocyte sedimentation rate (ESR)
    rebuck skin window technique
    chemotactic assay
  2. Tests of phagocytic function
    phagocytic index
    bactericidal activity
    NBT test
    WBC enzymes
B. Specific immune response tests
  1. Enumeration of B and T lymphocytes
    EA ⎫
    EAC ⎬ Rosettes
    E ⎭
  2. Tests of humoral function
    immunoglobulin levels
    specific antibody responses (IgM, IgG)
    Shick and Dick tests (IgG)
  3. Tests of cell-mediated function
	skin tests
	Candida
	SKSD
	DNCB
	skin grafts
	lymphocyte stimulation: PHA, antigen
	measurement of effector molecules (MIF)
	C. Tissue-damaging immune response
	  1. Tests of IgE hypersensitivity
	    RIST, PRIST, RAST
	    immediate hypersensitivity skin tests
	    histamine release
	  2. Tests of cytotoxic injury
	    red cells agglutinins
	    Coombs'
	  3. Tests of antigen-antibody complex injury
	    rheumatoid factor
	    antinuclear factor or LE prep
	    serum complement
	    tissue biopsy
	  4. Tests of injury due to delayed hypersensitivity
	    tissue biopsy
	    skin tests

Note: Not all inclusive.

1. Red blood cell (RBC) count is an actual count of circulating RBC in 1 cu mm of venous blood. When the RBC count is decreased by greater than ten percent of normal, it usually indicates anemia. It also can indicate a recent hemorrhage, hemolysis, dietary deficiency, genetic aberrations, drug ingestion, e.g., chloramphenicol, marrow failure, or chronic illness. An elevated RBC count may be seen in high altitudes or chronic hypoxia as a result of the body's requirements for greater oxygen carrying capacity.

2. Hemoglobin (Hgb) measures the total amount of Hbg in peripheral blood. Changes in plasma volume are more accurately reflected by

Hgb concentrations. Dilutional overhydration decreases the Hgb concentration whereas dehydration tends to cause an artificially high value.

3. Hematocrit (Hct) is the percentage of RBC in the total blood volume.

4. Mean corpuscular volume (MCV) is a measure of the average volume or the size of a single RBC. It is a useful measure in classifying anemias. It is derived by dividing the Hct by the total number of RBCs. When the MCV is elevated, the RBC is said to be macrocytic or abnormally large as seen in megaloblastic anemias. When the MCV is decreased, the RBC is abnormally small or microcytic as seen in iron deficiency anemia or thalassemia.

5. Mean corpuscular hemoglobin (MCH) measures the average amount of Hgb in an RBC. It is derived by dividing the Hgb concentration by the number of RBCs. Because macrocytic cells generally have more Hgb and microcytic cells generally have less, the causes for abnormal values closely resemble those for MCV.

6. Mean corpuscular Hgb concentration (MCHC) is a measure of the average concentration or percentage of Hgb in a single RBC. It is derived by dividing the Hgb by the hematocrit. When MCHC is decreased, the cell has a deficiency of Hgb and is hypochromic as in iron deficiency and thalassemia. Because RBCs cannot contain more Hgb than is physiologically possible, elevated MCHC values cannot occur, even when MCV levels are increased.

   When one investigates the causes of an anemia, it is helpful to categorize the anemia according to the RBC indices as follows:
   Normocytic, normochromic anemia
   > Chronic illness
   > Acute blood loss
   > Aplastic anemia
   > Acquired hemolytic anemias as in malfunctioning prosthetic cardiac valves
   Microcytic, hypochromic
   > Iron deficiency
   > Thalassemia
   > Lead poisoning
   Microcytic, normochromic
   > Renal disease
   Macrocytic, normochromic
   > Vitamin B_{12} or folic acid deficiency
   > Hydantoin ingestion

7. Differential is a measure of the total number of white blood cells (WBC) and the percentages of the five types of WBC. An increased total WBC count, leukocytosis, usually indicates infection or leukemia. Trauma or stress, either emotional or physical, can elevate the WBC count. Leukopenia, or a decreased WBC count, occurs in many forms

of bone marrow failure such as after antineoplastic therapy or in agranulocytosis, overwhelming infectons, dietary deficiency, and autoimmune diseases.

Neutrophils, called band cells in their immature stage of development, are the leukocytes responsible for phagocytosis. Elevations of any one type of WBC may indicate a specific disease. Increased neutrophils, neutrophilia, may indicate physical or emotional stress, acute infections, myelocytic leukemia, trauma, or ketoacidosis. A decreased neutrophil count, neutropenia, may indicate aplastic anemia, use of myelotoxic drugs as in chemotherapy, dietary deficiency, or overwhelming bacterial infection especially in the aged.

An increased lymphocyte count, or lymphocytosis, as indicative of chronic bacterial infection, viral infection, lymphocytic leukemia, multiple myeloma, or infectious mononucleosis. A decreased lymphocyte count may indicate leukemia, use of antineoplastic drugs, sepsis, or immune deficiency diseases.

Elevated eosinophil counts are indicative of parasitic infection, allergic reactions, eczema, leukemia, or autoimmune diseases. Decreased eosinophil counts may indicate increased adrenal steroid production.

Reticulocyte Count (Retic Count). This is a test for determining bone marrow function. A reticulocyte is an immature RBC and the retic count represents a direct measurement of RBC production by the bone marrow. Increased lymphocyte counts are expected as physiologic compensation in clients who are anemic. A normal or low retic count in an anemic client indicates that the marrow production of RBC is inadequate and is perhaps the cause of the anemia.

An elevated retic count in clients with a normal CBC indicates RBC overproduction (polycythemia vera). To determine if the elevated retic count is reflective of an adequate erythropoiesis in an anemic client with a low Hct, one can determine the retic index as follows:

$$\text{retic index} - \frac{\text{retic count (in \%)}\ \ \frac{\text{Hct}}{\text{normal Hct}}}{}$$

The retic index in a client who has a good marrow response to the anemia should be 1. If it is below 1, even though the reti count is increased in the anemic client, the blone marrow response is inadequate in its ability to compensate.

Iron Level with Total Iron Binding Capacity Test (Fe and TIBC). Abnormal levels of irons and total iron binding capacity are characteristic of many diseases including iron deficiency anemias. Serum iron determination is a measurement of the quantity of iron bound to transferrin. TIBC is a direct, quantitative measurement of transferrin.

Iron deficiency anemia has many causes including:

- insufficient iron intake
- inadequate gut absorption
- increased requirements
- loss of blood

Iron deficiency results in a decreased production of Hgb, which in turn results in a small, pale RBC—microcytic, hypochromic.

Chronic illness, e.g., infection or neoplasia, is characterized by low serum iron level and a decrease in iron binding capacity. Because iron requirements are high in pregnancy, it is not unusual to find low serum iron levels and high TIBC in late pregnancy.

Serum Haptoglobin Test. This test is used to detect intravascular destruction (hemolysis) of RBCs. Haptoglobins are glycoproteins produced by the liver and are Hgb-binding proteins. In hemolytic anemias associated with intravascular destruction of RBCs, the released Hgb is quickly bound to haptoglobin and the new complex quickly catabolized. This causes a marked decrease of the amount of free haptoglobin in the serum, which cannot be quickly compensated for by normal liver production. As a result, the client demonstrates a transient reduced level of haptoglobin.

Serum haptoglobins are decreased also in primary liver disease unassociated with hemolytic anemias. It is elevated in many inflammatory diseases.

Bone Marrow Examination. A normal bone marrow examination reveals active erythroid cell, myeloid cell, and megakaryocyte (platelet) production. It is performed to fully evaluate hematopoiesis. Examination of the bone marrow reveals the number, size, and shape of the RBC, WBC, and megakaryocytes as these cells evolve through various stages of development.

Samples of bone marrow can be obtained by aspiration or surgical removal from the sternum, iliac crest, iliac spines, and proximal fibia (in children). Microscopic examination includes an estimation of cellularity, determination of the presence of fibrotic tissue or neoplasms, and estimation of iron storage.

For estimation of cellularity, the specimen is examined and the relative quantity of each cell type is determined. Leukemias or leukemoid reactions are suspected when increased numbers of leukocyte precursors are present. Physiologic marrow compensation for infection is also recognized by an increased number of leukocyte precursors. Decreased numbers of marrow leukocyte precursors occur in clients with myelofibrosis, old age, metastatic neoplasia, or agranulocytosis, and after chemotherapy or radiation therapy.

Increased number of marrow RBC precursors occur with polycythemia vera or as a physiologic compensation to hemorrhagic or hemolytic anemias. Decreased numbers of marrow RBC precursors occur with erythroid hypoplasia following chemotherapy or radiation therapy, administration of other toxic drugs, or marrow replacement by fibrotic tissue or neoplasms.

Increased number of platelet precursors are seen in the marrow of clients following acute hemorrhage or some forms of chronic myeloid leukemia. This increase may also be compensatory in clients with secondary hypersplenism associated with portal hypertension or other conditions. Decreased megakaryocytes occur in clients who have had radiation therapy or chemotherapy and in clients with neoplastic or fibrotic marrow infiltrative diseases and aplastic anemias.

Lymphocyte precursors are increased in infections, lymphocytic leukemia, and lymphoma. Plasma cells are increased in clients with multiple myelomas, Hodgkin's disease, hypersensitivity states, rheumatic fever, and other chronic inflamatory diseases.

Estimation of cellularity can also be expressed as a ratio of myeloid WBC to erythroid RBC cells. The normal M:E (myeloid:erythroid) ratio is about 3:1. The M:E ratio is greater than normal in those diseases mentioned above in which increased leukocyte precursors are present or in which there is a decrease in erythroid precursors. The M:E ratio is less than normal when either leukocyte precursors are decreased or erythroid precursors are increased.

Drug induced or idiopathic myelofibrosis can be detected by examination of the bone marrow. With the use of special stains, iron stores can be estimated by the marrow biopsy. Leukemias, multiple myelomas, and polycythemia vera can easily be detected in biopsy specimens.

Hemoglobin Electrophoresis. This test enables one to detect abnormal forms of Hgb (hemoglobinopathies). Although many different Hgb variations have been described, the more common types are A_1, A_2, F, S, and C. Each major Hgb type is charged to varying degrees. When placed in an electromagnetic field, the Hgb variants migrate at different rates and therefore spread apart from each other. One is able to quantitate each band as a percentage of the total Hgb.

Hgb A_1 constitutes the major component of Hgb in the normal RBC. Hgb A_2 is only a minor component (2 to 3 percent). Hgb F is the major Hgb in the fetus yet exists in only minimal quantities in the normal adult. Levels of Hgb F greater than 2 percent in clients over 3 years old are abnormal. Hgb F is able to transport oxygen (O_2) when only small amounts of O_2 are available (as in fetal life). In clients requiring compensation for prolonged chronic hypoxia, for instance with congenital cardiac abnormalities, Hgb F increases to assist in the transport of the available O_2. Clients with hemoglobinopathies who are incapable of transporting adequate amounts of O_2, e.g., thalassemia, also show increased levels of Hgb F as a compensation.

Hgb S is an abnormal form of Hgb that is associated with sickle cell anemia, which occurs in American blacks. Hgb S is a relatively insoluble variant. When little O_2 is available, it assumes a crescent (sickle-type) shape that greatly distorts the RBC morphology. Vascular sludging is a consequence of the localized sickling and may lead to organ infarction.

Hgb C is another Hgb variant found in American blacks. RBCs containing Hgb C have a short life span and are more readily lysed than normal RBCs. Mild hemolytic anemia may result.

Peripheral Blood Smear. A smear of peripheral blood is the most informative of all hematological tests. All three hematological cell lines can be examined. Microscopic examination of RBCs can reveal variation in size (anisocytosis), shape (poikilocytosis), color, or intracellular content.

Classification of RBCs according to these variables is most helpful in identifying the causes of anemia.

1. RBC size
    Microcytes are small RBCs and indicate iron deficiency, hereditary spherocytosis, or thalassemia. Macrocytes are large RBCs and are seen in vitamin B_{12} or folic acid deficiency, reticulocytosis due to accelerated erythropoiesis, liver disorders, or postsplenectomy anemia.
2. RBC shape
    Spherocytes are small, round RBCs and are seen in hereditary spherocytosis and acquired immunohemolytic anemia. Elliptocytes are elliptical in shape and are seen in hereditary elliptocytosis and sickle cell anemia. Leptocytes, or target cells, are thin with small amounts of Hgb and are indicative of hemoglobinopathies and thalassemia. Spicule cells are seen in uremia, liver disease, and bleeding ulcers.
3. RBC color
    Hypochromic RBCs are pale and are seen in iron deficiency, thalassemia, and cardiac disease. Hyperchromasia is seen in dehydration due to the overconcentration of Hgb.
4. RBC intracellular structure
    a. Nucleus
        Because the maturation process of RBCs results in the loss of the nucleus, nucleated RBCs (normoblasts) seen in a peripheral blood smear indicate accelerated RBC production. It is a physiologic response to an RBC deficiency, hypoxemia, marrow-occupying neoplasm, or fibrotic tissue.
    b. Basophilic stippling
        These bodies are enclosed or included in the RBC. It is seen in lead poisoning and reticulocytosis.
    c. Howell-Jolly bodies
        These bodies are small, round remnants of nuclear material. They are seen postsplenectomy, in hemolytic anemia, and megaboblastic anemia.
    d. Heinz bodies
        These bodies are small, irregular particles of Hgb and are seen in drug-induced RBC injury, hemoglobinopathies, and hemolytic anemias.

Sickle Cell Test. Sickle cell disease and sickle cell trait can be detected by this study. Routine peripheral blood of clients with sickle cell disease does not contain sickled RBCs unless hypoxemia is present. In the sickle cell test, a deoxygenating agent is added to the person's blood. If 25 percent or more of the client's Hgb is of the S variation, the cells assume the crescent shape and the test is positive.

Direct Coombs' Test. This is a test to detect antibodies against RBC. Many diseases such as erythroblastosis fetalis, lymphomas, lupus, mycoplasmal infections, mononucleosis along with drugs (alpha methyldopa, levodopa, penicillin, and quinidine) are associated with production of antibodies. These antibodies result in hemolytic anemia. Frequently, the production of these autoantibodies against RBCs is not associated with any specific disease and the resulting hemolytic anemia is called idiopathic. The test is performed by mixing the client's RBCs, which are suspected of being covered with autoantibodies against RBCs, with Coombs' serum. Coombs' serum is a solution containing antibodies against human blood serum. If the RBCs are coated with autoantibodies against RBCs, the Coombs' antibodies will react with the antibodies on the RBCs, and cause agglutination of the RBCs. The greater the quantity of antibodies against RBCs present, the more clumping will occur. This test is read as positive with clumping on a scale of trace to $+4$.

When a transfusion with incompatible blood is given, the Coombs' test can detect the antibodies coating the transfused RBCs. This test is therefore very helpful in evaluating suspected transfusion reactions.

Indirect Coombs' Test. This study detects the presence of circulating antibodies against RBCs. The major purpose of this test is to determine if the client has serum antibodies (other than the major ABO system) to RBCs that he is about to receive by blood transfusion. A small amount of the recipient's serum is added to the donor's RBCs. Then Coombs' serum is added to the mixture. Visible agglutination indicates that the recipient has antibodies to the donor's RBCs. Therefore agglutination occurs when the antibodies against human serum in the Coombs' serum react with the recipient's antibodies that have coated the donor's RBC.

Circulating antibodies against RBCs may also occur in a pregnant woman who is Rh negative and is carrying an Rh positive fetus.

Blood Typing. By this test, ABO and Rh antigens can be detected on the blood of prospective blood donors and potential blood recipients. Human blood is grouped according to the presence or absence of these antigens. The two major antigens, A and B, form the basis of the ABO system. Group A RBCs contain A antigens; group B RBCs contain B antigens; group AB RBCs have both A and B antigens; and group O RBCs have neither A nor B antigens. The presence or absence of Rh antigens on the RBCs determines the classifications of Rh positive or negative.

There are many potential minor antigens not routinely detected during blood typing. If allowed to go unrecognized, these minor antigens can also initiate a blood transfusion reaction. Therefore, blood is not only typed but also cross matched to identify a mismatch of blood caused by minor antigens. Cross matching consists of the mixing the recipient's serum with the donor's RBCs in saline followed by the addition of Coombs' serum.

Coagulation Tests

Prothrombin Time (PT) Test. This test is used to evaluate the adequacy of the extrinsic coagulation system and the common pathway in the clotting mechanism. When the clotting factors, especially factors V and VII, exist in deficient quantities the PT is prolonged. Many diseases and drugs are associated with decreased levels of these factors. These include:

1. Hepatocellular liver disease (cirrhosis, hepatitis, and cancer). Factors II, VII, IX, and X are produced in the liver. With severe hepatocellular dysfunction, this synthesis will not occur and serum concentration of these factors will be decreased. Even a small decrease in factor VII will result in marked prolongation of the PT.
2. Obstructive biliary disease, e.g., bile duct obstruction due to tumors, stones, or intrahepatic cholestasis which may be due to sepsis or drugs. Without the bile necessary for fat absorption, fat malabsorption occurs in the gut and vitamins A, D, E, and K are not absorbed. Because synthesis of factors II, VII, IX, and X are dependent on vitamin K, these factors will not be adequately produced. Factor VII is the first to decrease and will result in prolongation of PT.

   Parenchymal liver disease can be differentiated from obstructive biliary disease by a determination of the client's response to parenteral vitamin K administration. If the PT returns to normal after 3 days of vitamin K administration, the client has obstructive biliary disease which led to vitamin K malabsorption. If it does not return to normal, severe hepatocellular disease exists and liver cells are incapable of synthesizing the clotting factors.
3. Coumarin ingestion. Coumarin is used to prevent coagulation in clients with thromboembolic disease. These drugs interfere with the production of vitamin K-dependent clotting factors and result in a prolongation of the PT. Adequacy of coumarin therapy can be monitored by following the PT. Appropriate coumarin therapy should prolong the PT by 1½ to 2 times the control (or 20 to 30 percent of the normal value).

The PT test results are usually given in seconds along with a control value. The control usually varies somewhat from day to day because of reagents used. The client's PT should be about equal to the control value. Some laboratories report PT values or percentages of normal activity, or the client's results are compared with a curve representing normal clotting time. A client receiving anticoagulants should be within a therapeutic range of 20 to 30 percent.

Partial Prothrombin Time (PTT) Test. The PTT is used to assess the intrinsic system and the common pathway of clot formation. It evaluates factors II, V, VII, IX, XI, and XII. When any of these factors exists in inadequate quantities, as in hemophilia A and B or consumptive coagulopathy, the PTT is prolonged. Because factors II, IX, and X are vitamin K-dependent factors produced in the liver, hepatocellular disease or biliary obstruction can decrease their concentration and thus prolong the PTT.

Heparin inactivates prothrombin and prevents formation of thromboplastin. These actions prolong the intrinsic clotting pathway for 4 to 6 hours after each dose of heparin. The appropriate dose of heparin can be monitored by PTT. The PTT test results are given in seconds along with a control. The control value may vary slightly from day to day because of reagents used. Recently, activators have been added to the PTT test reagents to shorten normal clotting time and provide a narrow normal range. This shortened time is called the activated partial thromboplastin time (APTT). A normal APTT is 30 to 40 seconds. Desired ranges for therapeutic anticoagulation are 1½ to 2½ times normal. The specimen should be drawn 30 to 60 minutes before the client's next heparin dose is given. If the APTT is less than 60 seconds, the client is not receiving therapeutic anticoagulation and needs more heparin. An APTT of more than 100 seconds indicates too much heparin is being given and a risk of serious spontaneous bleeding exists.

Platelet Count. This is an actual count of the number of platelets. Because platelets can clump together, automated counting is subject to at least a 10 to 15 percent error. Counts of less than 100,000 are considered thrombocytopenia. Thrombocytosis is said to exist when counts are more than 400,000. Spontaneous bleeding is a serious danger when counts are less than 15,000. With counts of more than 40,000, spontaneous bleeding rarely occurs. However, prolonged bleeding from trauma or surgery may occur at this level. Causes of thrombocytopenia include:

- decreased production (bone marrow failure or infiltration)
- sequestration (hypersplenism)
- accelerated destruction of platelets (antibodies, infections, prosthetic heart valves)
- consumption [disseminated intravascular coagulation (DIC)], and
- platelet loss from hemorrhage.

Thrombocytosis may occur as a compensatory response to severe hemorrhage. Other conditions associated with it are polycythemia vera, leukemia, postsplenectomy syndromes, and various malignant disorders. Vascular thrombosis with organ infarction is the only major complication of thrombocytosis.

TABLE 1-2. COAGULATION FACTORS IN BLOOD PRODUCTS

Factor	Minimum Hemostatic Level in mg/dl	Blood Component
I	60–100	C, FFP, FWB
II	10–15	P, WB, FFP, FWB
V	5–10	FFP, FWB
VII	5–20	P, WB, FFP, FWB
VIII	30	C, FFP, VIII conc
IX	30	FFP, FWP
X	8–10	P, WB, FFP, FWB
XI	25	P, WB, FFP, FWB

C = cryoprecipitate; FWB = whole blood less than 24° old; P = unfrozen banked plasma; WB = whole blood, banked; VIII conc = factor VIII concentrate.

Bleeding Time Test. This test is used to evaluate the vascular and platelet factors associated with hemostasis. For this study, a small incision is made in the forearm, and the time required for the bleeding to stop is recorded. Prolonged values may be due to deficient platelet production, infiltration of marrow, platelet consumption, increased platelet destruction, inadequate platelet function caused by aspirin or von Willebrand's disease, increased capillary fragility due to collagen vascular disease or Henoch-Schönlein syndrome, or ingestion of antiinflammatory drugs.

Coagulation Factors Concentration Test. This test is a measure of the concentration of a specific coagulation factor in the blood. Testing is now available to measure the quantity of factors I, II, V, VII, VIII, IX, X, and XI. When these factors exist in concentrations less than the minimum hemostatic level, the clotting time is prolonged. These minimal hemostatic levels vary according to the factor involved (Tables 1–2 and 1–3).

Euglobin Lysis Time Test. This test is a measure of the activity of systemic fibrinolysis. Fibrin, found in the euglobin fraction of plasma, is normally very

TABLE 1-3. CONDITIONS THAT MAY RESULT IN COAGULATION FACTOR DEFICIENCY

Disease	Factors Affected
Liver disease	I, II, V, VII, IX, X, XI
DIC	I, V, VIII
Fibrinolysis	I, V, VIII
Congenital deficiency	I, II, V, VII, VIII, IX, X, XI
Heparin administration	II
Warfarin ingestin	II, VII, IX, X, XI
Autoimmune disease	VIII

rapidly dissolved by plasmin. The time measured from clot formation to clot lysis is the euglobin lysis time. In primary fibrinolysis, seen in streptokinase administration, cancer of the prostate, or shock, the euglobin lysis time is short. In DIC, euglobin lysis time is usually normal. If all of the plasmin has been consumed, however, the time may be prolonged. This is one of the best tests used to differentiate primary fibrinolysis from DIC. This differentiation is important in considering appropriate therapy for the client with a bleeding tendency. Epsilon aminocaproic acid may be required to treat primary fibrinolysis; heparin may be indicated for DIC. This test may also be used to monitor streptokinase or urokinase therapy.

Fibrin Degradation Products (FDP) Test. This test provides a direct indication of the activity of the fibrinolytic system. When plasma acts to dissolve fibrin clots, fibrinogen and FDPs are formed and these degradation products can be measured. When they are present in large amounts, they indicate increased fibrinolysis as it occurs in DIC and primary fibrinolytic disorders.

Immunological System
The tests that may be used in assessing immunological function are classified in three categories: nonspecific, specific, and tissue damaging immune responses.

Nonspecific Tests. These tests measure one or more aspects of the inflammatory response and phagocytosis. They include: WBC count and differential, sedimentation rate, C-reactive protein, complement activity, Rebuck skin window technique, and chemotactic assay. These tests are all useful in assessing whether an inflammatory response is in progress and in determining the functional integrity of the afferent limb of the immune response. In general, they are all increased during the phase of acute inflammation, and the sedimentation rate is elevated in more protracted (chronic) inflammatory responses.

Complement activity measurement is a useful test in several clinical situations. Either total serum complement or individual complement components may be measured. C_3 is the major component of the complement in serum and is easily measured by radial immunodiffusion. The complement system is evaluated to detect deficiencies resulting from inborn deficiencies of the complement components or increased complement utilization resulting from ongoing immunological processes.

PHAGOCYTIC FUNCTION. These tests of phagocytosis measure the capacity of the phagocytic cells to take up inert particles. They include: phagocytic index, bactericidal activity, quantitative NBT test, and measurement of specific WBC enzymes. Tests of phagocytosis are performed in clients suspected of having disorders of the phagocytes.

Specific Tests. Tests of specific immune function measure those functions associated with humoral immunity or with cellular immunity.

1. Enumeration of B and T lymphocytes. This is a test to determine relative numbers of B and T lymphocytes. The commonly measured lymphocyte markers are EA, EAC, and E rosettes. Clinical indications for enumeration of lymphocyte subpopulations include lymphoproliferative disease, immune deficiency disease, and immunologically mediated disease.

2. Tests of humoral function include quantification of immunoglobulins; specific antibody responses, e.g., isohemagglutinins; Shick and Dick tests; and specific antibody responses.

3. Tests for cellular immune function include skin tests, e.g., *Candida*, DNCB; lymphocyte stimulation; and measurement of effector molecules.

Tissue Damaging Immune Response Tests. Tests of tissue damaging immune function measure immune responses that cause disease manifestations through immunological injury. These tests include: measurement of IgE by immediate hypersensitivity skin testing; Coombs' test; rheumatoid factor; and lupus erythematosus cell phenomenon and tissue biopsy. These are indicated when manifestations of immunologically mediated diseases are present.

Nursing Diagnosis

Nursing diagnosis is an integral part of the nursing process. Diagnoses are made for the purpose of planning care. Nursing diagnoses, or clinical diagnoses made by professional nurses, describe actual or potential health problems that nurses by virtue of their education and experience are able and legally responsible, accountable, and licensed to treat. Nursing diagnosis is a statement that describes a health state or an actual or potential alteration in one's life processes (physiological, psychological, sociocultural, developmental, and spiritual). The nurse uses the nursing process to identify and synthesize clinical data and to order nursing interventions to reduce, eliminate, or prevent (health promotion) health alterations that are in the legal and educational domain of nursing.

The accepted diagnoses to date are limited. Nursing diagnoses are still in a developmental stage. Hopefully, this will not prevent practitioners from using them. Diagnoses need to be identified and validated in the clinical setting. Presently there are many client situations and problems that are not covered by the accepted diagnoses. Practitioners should develop their own diagnoses and submit them for discussion to the North American Nursing Diagnosis Association. Therefore, throughout this book, nursing diagnoses will be used that are not presently in the accepted list.

The diagnostic statement should be a two-part statement consisting of the diagnostic title linked with the etiological and contributing factors. An example is alteration in bowel elimination: constipation related to immobility secondary to traction. The use of the words "related to" reflects a relationship between the first and second parts of the statement. It is important that the nurse not link the statements with words implying cause–effect because such a relationship can result in legal or professional difficulty. Using a diagnostic label by itself without "related to" etiological or contributing factor would result in a vaguely stated problem that is not specific enough to direct individualized interventions. The more specific the second part of the statement the more specialized the interventions can be. The linking of the diagnostic category with contributing factors also assists the nurse in validating the category. If the defining characteristics of a diagnostic category are present but the etiological with contributing factors are unknown, the statement can be written as: Ineffective family coping: manifested by anger at staff related to unknown etiology.

Nursing Interventions

Goals for nursing interventions are written to direct care, to identify desired outcomes, and to measure the effectiveness of the interventions. Nursing orders follow the goals. The nurse focuses on prescribing the care required to prevent, reduce, or eliminate the alteration. The objective of the nursing order is to direct individualized care to a client.

Evaluation

Evaluation is the final component of the nursing process. It consists of three distinct activities.

1. Establishing criteria to observe and measure.
2. Assessing present response for evidence.
3. Comparing present response to the established criteria.

SUMMARY

Of course, one cannot begin to identify problems or plan nursing care without a sound base in the physiology and pathophysiology of that system. The following three chapters are essential to the full comprehension of the remainder of the text.

CHAPTER 2
Physiology of the Hematopoietic System

BLOOD FORMING ORGANS

Bone Marrow

A reasonable place to begin a discussion of hematopoietic physiology is the bone marrow. It is the production site of the cellular elements of the blood: erythroid, myeloid, and thrombocytic. In addition, it is one source of lymphocytes and macrophages. The bone marrow is involved in antigen processing, cellular and humoral immunity, and recognition and removal of senescent cells.

In the fetus, hematopoiesis, or blood cell production, begins in the liver and the yolk sac. By the twentieth week of fetal life, it occurs in the bone marrow. By the thirtieth week, the bone marrow has achieved full cellularity. Fetal hematopoiesis also occurs in the liver, spleen, lymph nodes, and thymus. At birth hematopoiesis occurs in almost every bone. The flat bones—sternum, ribs, skull, pelvic, and shoulder girdles, vertebrae, and innominates—retain most of their hematopoietic activity throughout life. Hematopoiesis gradually decreases within the shafts of the long bones, however, and in the adult, it is limited to the ends of the long bones. By age 18, normal adult distribution of marrow is established and the gradual cessation of hematopoiesis leads to replacement of inactive bone marrow by fatty tissue. Later in life, the proportion of fatty marrow increases so that in old age it occupies about half of the ribs and the sternum. At times of increased demand for blood cells, active marrow can reappear in any of these sites.

Stem Cells

How does the bone marrow "create" the needed cells? It contains pluripotent stem cells—cells that give rise to the several lines of differentiated blood cells and are self-maintaining. A pluripotent stem cell (or colony forming unit, CFU) is uncommitted. It can differentiate into an erythroid, granulocytic, thrombocytic, or lymphoid cell line. The pluripotent stem cells are small and mononuclear, resemble lymphocytes, are few in number, mobile, and are normally present in the blood. At the times of increased demand, the number can increase. For example, after whole body irradiation, the number of stem cells in blood increases. Clinically, this results in a marked increase in cell development and restoration of the bone marrow to normal.

The next stage in cell development is the committed, or unipotential, stem cells. They are also called precursor cells, progenitor cells, or early differentiated cells. These are cells with little or no self-replicating capacity but are sensitive to specific regulatory factors and are capable of differentiating into one cell line. Each cell line has its own specific unipotential stem cell, one for lymphocytes, one for granulocytes and macrophages, one for erythrocytes, and one for platelets.

Unipotential stem cells are in active cell cycle and are capable of self-renewal for a considerable period of time. However, they need a stimulus to get going. A humoral poietin is required before the cell becomes further differentiated. Erythropoietin is specific for stem cells committed to erythropoiesis, but there is mounting evidence of the existence of a leukopoietin and a thrombopoietin (Fig. 2–1).

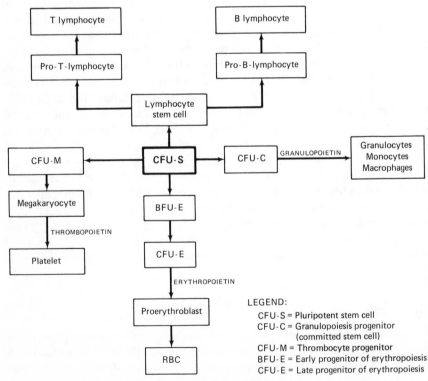

Figure 2-1. Cellular development.

Spleen

The spleen is beneath the diaphragm, behind and to the left of the stomach. Although not essential for life, it performs many important functions. The spleen contains both lymphoid and reticuloendothelial elements. It comprises the largest collection of lymphocytes and reticuloendothelial cells in the body, and plays an active part in antibody synthesis and other defense mechanisms.

There are three types of pulp within the spleen: white, red, and marginal pulp. White pulp is packed with lymphocytes and free macrophages. Red pulp is a mass of vascular sinuses lined by reticuloendothelial cells that phagocytize and remove unwanted cells from the bloodstream. Many arteries terminate within the marginal pulp. The spleen has seven functions:

1. In fetal life, it is important in hematopoiesis. In early life, lymphocytes leave the thymus and colonize the spleen and the lymph nodes. Lymphocytes found in the adult spleen are partly descendants of these original thymus lymphocytes and partly sequestered blood borne lymphocytes.

2. Culling function, or hemoclastic function, describes the spleen's ability to destroy aged or imperfect red blood cells (RBCs) by phagocytosis.

3. Pitting function is the spleen's ability to remove particles from intact RBCs without destroying them. These particles, for example Howell-Jolly or Heinz bodies, are pinched off because they are having difficulty squeezing through the splenic circulation.

4. Reservoir function describes the spleen's ability to serve as a storage area for platelets. Twenty to thirty percent of the platelet mass is sequestered in the spleen. With splenomegaly, up to 30 percent of the RBC mass and 80 to 90 percent of the platelet mass may be stored in the spleen.

5. The spleen serves as a compartmental structure. It plays a major role in removing effete RBCs from the circulation. When blood enters the red pulp, it must navigate the circuitous and macrophage-lined compartments before penetrating the narrow holes through which it gains access into the spleen. In traversing this pathway to the spleen, blood is brought into intimate contact with the phagocytic reticuloendothelial cells of the white, marginal, and red pulp.

6. The spleen also plays a part in iron metabolism. The reticuloendothelial cells catabolize hemoglobin released from those RBCs that have been destroyed in the spleen. Iron is then returned to the bone marrow for reuse.

7. The spleen serves as both a mechanical filter and an early source of antibody activity. Clients who have had splenectomies as a result of traumatic injuries, cancer treatment, or other diseases have a greatly increased risk of sepsis and death. Splenectomized clients maintain diminished antibody activity when challenged with particulate antigens; are deficient in tuft sin, the phagocytosis-promoting peptide;

and have decreased levels of IgM and properdin. Consequently, splenectomized clients are at increased risk for septicemia, usually with *staphylococcus pneumonia, Neisseria meningitis,* or *Hemophilus influenza.* Septicemia is usually fulminant with a large number of organisms in the bloodstream and can occur days to years after a splenectomy. Death due to sepsis in splenectomized individuals was calculated to occur 200 times more frequently than in the general population. Although the incidence of postsplenectomy septicemia is especially significant in children and adolescents also receiving chemotherapy, bacteremia can occur even when clients are not granulocytopenic, suggesting that splenectomy is an important independent risk factor for cancer patients. Splenectomy does not appear to enhance the risk for most nonbacterial infections, e.g., herpes zoster.

The splenectomized client is unable to dispose of blood borne pyogenic organisms because such organisms are often encapsulated and resistant to phagocytosis, and the client lacks the normal phagocytic activity of clearing small amounts of encapsulated matter from the blood. The spleen is an early source of opsonin activity, or the process by which foreign material is prepared for phagocytosis. Opsonins increase the specific rate of bacterial ingestion by phagocytes after binding to the surface of bacteria. Opsonins are therefore of primary importance in defense against pyrogenic pathogens. Because the client lacks opsonins, the unimpeded organism population can double every 20 to 40 minutes. Under these circumstances, fulminant sepsis may develop rapidly. The splenectomized client should be observed constantly for sepsis and all infections should be treated promptly and vigorously. Pneumococcal vaccines, currently under investigation, may provide some protection for these clients.

Liver

The liver forms a large proportion of blood substances used in the coagulation process. These include fibrinogen, prothrombin, accelerator globulin, and factors VII, IX, and X.

The liver will contribute to erythropoiesis if RBC production in the bone marrow is accelerated or abnormal, especially with ineffective erythropoiesis as in megaloblastic anemia. For example, under extreme and very prolonged stress or in the face of marrow replacement by cancer cells, the liver may develop foci of erythropoiesis.

The liver also converts bilirubin, which is the end product of hemoglobin decomposition, to bile, necessary for fat digestion. Bile production is increased by excessive RBC destruction, for instance in hemolytic anemia and ineffective erythropoiesis. Ineffective erythropoiesis is destruction of defective RBC precursors within the marrow, or soon after release into the peripheral blood.

It occurs in thalassemia, megaloblastic anemia, sideroblastic anemia, and erythroleukemia.

The liver also stores iron in the form of ferritin. Hepatic cells contain large amounts of a protein called apoferritin, which is capable of combining with iron to form ferritin.

FORMATION AND FUNCTION OF THE FORMED ELEMENTS IN THE BLOOD

Erythroid Cell System: Erythropoiesis

The erythroid cell system, or RBCs, comprises the population of circulating RBCs and their nucleated precursors located in the normal adult bone marrow. The total mass of RBCs is regulated within very narrow limits so that an adequate number of cells are always available to provide sufficient tissue oxygenation. This regulation is precise enough to prevent overconcentration of RBC that would impede blood flow through the capillaries. It is the process of erythropoiesis that maintains the circulating red cell mass within relatively narrow limits. The predominant control of erythropoiesis is mediated through alterations in tissue oxygen tension.

The normal RBC count is 4,500,000 to 5,500,000 cells. Any condition that causes the quantity of oxygen (O_2) transported to the tissue to decrease, ordinarily increases the rate of RBC production. Therefore, when a client becomes anemic secondary to hemorrhage, for instance, the bone marrow immediately begins to produce large quantities of RBCs. Also destruction of major portions of the bone marrow by any means, especially radiation therapy, leads to hyperplasia of the remaining marrow, thereby attempting to supply the increased demand for RBCs in the body. At very high altitudes where the quantity of O_2 is greatly decreased, insufficient O_2 is transported to the tissues, and RBCs are then produced so rapidly that their number in the blood is considerably increased.

Erythropoietin is a humoral agent that appears in the blood in response to tissue hypoxia. It acts on the bone marrow to increase the rate of RBC production. There is no direct response of the bone marrow to hypoxia. Instead, hypoxia stimulates RBC production only through erythropoietin. A decrease in tissue oxygen tension, specifically in the kidneys, is believed to lead to an increase in the activity of erythropoietin.

The precise mechanisms for formation of erythropoietin is not clearly understood but it is known that only minute quantities of it are formed in persons whose kidneys have been removed. However, it has yet to be isolated from the kidneys. Small amounts are produced by extrarenal tissues as demonstrated in anephric animals and clients whose erythropoietin levels still rise in response to hypoxia. It is clear that other tissues, probably the liver, can form very slight amounts of the erythropoietic factor that lead to the formation of erythropoietin. Even so, in the absence of a kidney, a person usually becomes very anemic because of extremely low levels of circulating erythropoietin.

At present, it is believed that when the kidneys become hypoxic they release an enzyme called the renal erythropoietic factor, or erythrogeinen. It is secreted into the blood where its acts within minutes to isolate the erythropoietin molecule. Erythropoietin circulates in the blood for about a day and during this time acts on the bone marrow to cause erythropoiesis.

Erythropoietin is formed almost immediately after placing a person in a low oxygen atmosphere. There are no new RBCs in the blood within the first 2 days, but after 5 days a maximum amount of new RBCs is reached. Cells continue to be produced at this rate as long as the client remains in a low oxygen state, or until he has produced enough RBC to carry adequate amounts of O_2 to his tissues. Upon removal of the person from a state of low O_2 tension, his rate of O_2 transport to the tissues rises above normal, which causes the rate of erythropoietin formation to decrease. His rate of RBC production falls essentially to zero within several days. Cellular production remains at this level until enough cells have lived out their life span so tissues receive only their normal complement of O_2.

Erythropoietin is found in both plasma and urine, and levels bear an inverse relationship to hemoglobin (Hgb) levels. With chronic hypoxemia due to high altitudes, chronic obstructive pulmonary disease, or right to left shunts, an increased number of RBCs, or polycythemia, results from increased erythropoietin levels. Certain tumors are reported to be inappropriate producers of erythropoiesis-stimulating substances. Low levels of erythropoietin are found in a wide variety of chronic inflammatory disease and in renal failure. With stress, erythropoietin increases and rate of RBC production can rise to as high as six to eight times normal.

Red Blood Cells

The first recognizable developmental step in RBC life is the proerythroblast, which is the immediate descendant of the committed stem cell. The proerythroblast is also known as a pronormoblast, or hemocytoblast. One proerythroblast gives rise to 16 to 32 progeny erythrocytes. It is a nucleated cell and is in active synthesis of deoxyribonucleic acid (DNA), ribonucleic acid (RNA), and protein. Hemoglobin synthesis has not yet begun (Fig. 2–2).

The proerythroblast is succeeded by the basophilic erythroblast. There is a high concentration of cytoplasmic ribosomes present in this stage in preparation for the onset of Hgb synthesis (Table 2–1). The basophilic erythroblast is succeeded by the polychromatophilic erythroblast stage, which is characterized by initial Hgb synthesis. Cell division continues until the orthochromatic erythroblast stage is reached. At this point, the nucleus is expelled and the nuclear remnant is phagocytosed by macrophages. Hemoglobin synthesis continues on messenger RNA complexes. The reticulocyte is the next developmental

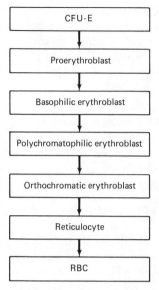

Figure 2-2. Red blood cells.

stage and is characterized by active hemoglobin synthesis. About 35 percent of Hgb synthesis occurs during this stage. At this point, the cells are released into the circulation. During the next 24 to 36 hours, the reticulocyte matures into the erythrocyte or RBC. The capacity for Hgb synthesis is lost, and the cell assumes its characteristic biconcave disk shape.

Normally, about 0.2 to 2 percent of circulating RBCs are reticulocytes because they survive as such for approximately 24 hours before maturing. About 1 percent of RBCs are replaced daily. The reticulocyte count is of particular importance because it is a parameter of RBC production rate. It is a good indicator of the erythropoietic response. It is elevated in most overt hemolytic anemias and may be absent in aplastic crises and in those with a primary cause, for instance chronic lymphocytic leukemia. Anemias without an appropriate reticulocytosis can occur if erythropoiesis is defective as in iron deficiency states and megaloblastic anemias.

TABLE 2-1. RED BLOOD CELL DEVELOPMENT

Stage in Development	Comments
Proerythroblast	Synthesis of DNA, RNA, protein
Basophilic erythroblast	Preparing for Hgb synthesis
Polychromatophilic erythroblast	Initial Hgb synthesis
Orthochromatic erythroblast	Nucleus expelled Hgb synthesis continues
Reticulocyte	Active Hgb synthesis
RBC	No capacity for Hgb synthesis

The normal erythrocyte is an extremely flexible and elastic biconcave disk without nuclei. It can travel at high speeds and can bend and twist as it passes through tiny capillaries. This ability to elongate exposes more of its surface area for exchange of O_2 and carbon dioxide (CO_2). Each milliliter of blood contains about 5 billion erythrocytes. The average life span of an RBC is 120 days.

The red cell membrane is composed of two components: the stroma, which is the innermost structure of the erythrocyte, and the outer cell membrane, which is the external portion of the erythrocyte. The membrane is composed of protein, lipid, and carbohydrate. Hemoglobin is attached to the stroma, and antigenic clusters are located on the outer cell membrane.

The RBC has the following functions:

1. To transport Hgb, which carries O_2 from the lungs to the tissues.
2. To catalyze the reaction between carbon dioxide and O_2, using carbonic anhydrase. By increasing the rapidity of this reaction, the RBCs make it possible for blood to react with large quantities of carbon dioxide and thereby transport it from the tissues to the lungs for excretion.
3. To contribute approximately 70 percent of all buffering power of whole blood.

Vitamin B_{12} (cobalamin) and folic acid are two vitamins essential for RBC synthesis. Deficiencies in these two vitamins can lead to maturational anemias.

Hemoglobin

The primary role of RBCs is to transport O_2 from the lungs to the tissues and to transport (CO_2) in the reverse direction. Both of these functions are accomplished through Hgb. About 98 percent of the protein in the cytoplasm of RBCs is Hgb. The Hgb molecule contains four hematology groups, one bound to each of four globin chains of Hgb. The hematology portion is synthesized from acetic acid and glycine, with synthesis occurring in the mitochondria. Acetic acid is changed, in the Krebs cycle, into a ketoglutaric acid. Two molecules of ketoglutaric acid combine with one molecule of glycine to form a pyrrole compound. Four pyrrole compounds combine to form a protoporphyrin compound, one of which combines with iron to form a hematologic molecule. Globin is a globulin that is synthesized in the endoplasmic reticulum, and is composed of four large polypeptide chains. The nature of these chains determines the binding affinity of Hgb for O_2, therefore, the Hgb molecule has four sites for attachment of O_2.

Embryonic hemoglobins are first recognized between 4 to 6 weeks of gestation. They are known as Gower I and Gower II. Later in fetal development, fetal hemoglobin, or Hgb F, is produced and is the major Hgb present at birth. It facilitates transfer of O_2 across the placenta. Hgb F is also present in the normal adult, as a minor component of adult Hgb. Hemoglobin A is the adult Hgb, and comprises about 97 percent of the total. The remaining 3 percent

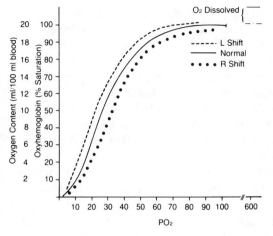

Figure 2-3. Oxyhemoglobin dissociation curve—expression of relationship between the percent saturation of hemoglobin with O_2 and the PO_2 of the plasma. *(From Guenter, C.A., & Welch, M. H., Pulmonary Medicine, Philadelphia, Lippincott, 1977.)*

is primarily Hgb A_2. Synthesis of Hgb A may begin in fetal life, but does not become the principle one in circulating RBC until after birth.

As has been noted earlier, Hgb is primarily responsible for O_2 transport. The diagram depicting the oxyhemoglobin dissociation curve (Fig. 2–3) is important because it demonstrates the considerable transfer of O_2 from Hgb to tissues with only a small drop in oxygen tension.

The oxyhemoglobin dissociation curve shows the progressive increase in the percentage of Hgb that is bound with O_2 as the PO_2 increases. This percentage is also known as the percent saturation of hemoglobin. One can see from the diagram that the usual O_2 saturation of arterial blood is 97 percent.

As arterial O_2 tension falls below 70 mm Hg, the curve becomes progressively steep; that is, the fall in saturation becomes progressively more rapid. Because of the steep slope of the dissociation curve, a small fall in PO_2 causes extreme amounts of O_2 to be released to the tissues. It is useful to remember that a PO_2 of 40, 50, and 60 mm Hg corresponds roughly to saturations of 70, 80, and 90 percent, respectively. This has direct implications for clinical practice. When a client is found to have a PO_2 of 60 mm Hg, his O_2 saturation is 90 percent. Therefore, if the nurse were to increase the amount of O_2 the client is receiving, the patient's PO_2 may increase but this would lead to only an insignificant rise in O_2 saturation. Because it is the O_2 saturation that reflects tissue oxygenation, increasing the client's PO_2 may only lead to an increased risk of O_2 toxicity.

A number of different factors can displace the dissociation curve in one direction or another. When the blood pH drops, the hemoglobin dissociation curve shifts to the right and more O_2 is then released to the tissues. On the other hand, an increase in pH shifts the curve to the left. Other factors that displace the curve to the right are increases in CO_2, blood temperature, and 2,3–DPG, a phosphate compound normally present in the blood. The normal

DPG in the blood keeps the hemoglobin dissociation curve shifted slightly to the right all of the time. However, in hypoxic conditions that last longer than a few hours, the quantity of DPG in the blood increases considerably, thus shifting the Hgb dissociation curve even farther to the right. This causes O_2 to be released to the tissues at as much as 10 mm Hg higher O_2 pressure than would be the case without the increased DPG. It has been thought that this might be an important mechanism for adaptation to hypoxia. However, the presence of the excess DPG also makes it difficult for the Hgb in the lungs to combine with oxygen in the hypoxia state, thereby often creating as much harm as good.

The shift of the Hgb dissociation curve by a change in blood CO_2 is important to enhance oxygenation of the blood in the lungs and also to enhance the release of O_2 from the blood in the tissues. This is the Bohr effect. As the blood passes through the lungs, CO_2 diffuses from the blood into the alveoli. This reduces the blood PCO_2 and increases the pH. Both of these effects shift the Hgb dissociation curve to the left. Therefore the quantity of O_2 that binds with Hgb becomes considerably increased and allows greater O_2 transport to the tissues. When the blood reaches the tissue capillaries, the opposite effect occurs. Carbon dioxide entering the blood from the tissues displaces O_2 from the Hgb and therefore delivers O_2 to the tissues at a higher PO_2 than would otherwise occur. That is, the dissociation curve shifts to the right in the tissues, exactly opposite to the leftward shift in the lungs.

Red Blood Cell Metabolism

Mature red cells consume little oxygen and do not synthesize protein. Glucose is the main metabolic substrate of red cells and is metabolized via two major pathways: the Embden-Meyerhof or glycolytic pathway and the hexosemonophosphate shunt pathway (HMP).

The Embden-Meyerhof pathway:

1. Metabolizes glucose to lactate (95 percent of glucose is metabolized to lactate via this pathway).
2. Synthesizes adenosine triphosphate (ATP), which contributes to active transport of sodium and potassium, maintenance of low intracellular calcium levels, and sustenance of glycolysis itself. Two moles of ATP are generated per mole of glucose consumed.
3. Is the major source of red cell NADH, which is an essential ingredient of many oxidation–reduction reactions.
4. Metabolizes 2,3–DPG.

The hexosemonophosphate shunt:

1. Is responsible for the metabolism of 5 to 10 percent of utilized glucose.
2. Produces NADPH, which is associated with glutathione metabolism.
3. Metabolizes glutathione. The tight coupling of HMP shunt and glutathione metabolism protects red cells from oxidant injury.

Many clinical problems can arise because of defects in the metabolic pathways. These clinical problems are discussed in a subsequent chapter.

Hemolysis

Red blood cells have a life span of 120 days. Most RBCs achieve a full life span indicating that red cells are destroyed by an age-dependent process. Age-dependent changes include decreased pliability of the membrane, accumulation of methemoglobin, or oxidation of cellular proteins. Senescent RBCs are selectively sequestered and destroyed by macrophages of the reticuloendothelial system. The spleen plays a predominant role in destruction of normally senescent red cells, although other reticuloendothelial organs, especially the liver, are competent to assume this. The signal that indicates a cell is ready for phagocytosis is not understood.

Within the macrophage, the cell is consumed by proteolytic and lipolytic enzymes. Much of the iron released from heme is reused for synthesis of new hemoglobin. The heme portion is converted into bilirubin by the reticuloendothelial system.

In a clinical sense, hemolysis refers to premature RBC destruction due to a number of factors. These clinical situations are discussed in subsequent chapters.

Varieties of Hemoglobin

There have been a number of Hgb variants identified to date. Many of these are due to genetic alterations, and often lead to hematologic disease. These diseases include sickle cell anemia and some hemolytic anemias. The thalassemias are a hereditary disorder of Hgb synthesis.

Methemoglobinemia is Hgb in which the iron has been oxidized, therefore this Hgb cannot carry O_2. Methemoglobin is continuously being formed in normal red cells, but under normal conditions is reduced to hemoglobin. Methemoglobinemia may develop when normal red cells are exposed to excess oxidant drugs or toxins, or it may be a congenital disorder. It leads to a progressive increase in oxygen affinity of the remaining functioning heme groups on the hemoglobin tetramer, causing a decrease in the amount of oxygen released to the tissues.

Leukocytic Cell System: Leukopoiesis

White Blood Cells

The circulating white blood cells (WBC) or leukocytes are of six types:

1. Polymorphonuclear neutrophils.
2. Polymorphonuclear eosinophils.
3. Polymorphonuclear basophils—the three "polymorphonuclear" types are granulocytes, because they have a granular appearance.
4. Monocytes/macrophages.

TABLE 2-2. LEUKOCYTES

WBC	Function
Neutrophils	Phagocytosis
Eosinophils	Allergic reactions
Basophils	Allergic reactions
Monocyte/Macrophage	Phagocytosis
Lymphocytes	Antibody production (B)
	Cellular immunity (T)
Plasma cell	Antibody production

    5. Lymphocytes.
    6. Plasma cells. (Table 2-2)

The WBCs are the mobile units of the body's protective system. They are formed partially in the bone marrow (granulocytes, monocytes, and a few lymphocytes), and partially in lymph tissues (lymphocytes and plasma cells). Leukopoiesis, or WBC development, is also thought to be influenced by chemicals resulting from dead or dying granulocytes, bacteria through the stimulus of chemotaxis, infection, androgen hormones, foreign substances, antibodies, and blood loss into body spaces.

In general, the granulocytes and the monocytes are responsible for phagocytosis, and the lymphocytes and plasma cells are responsible for antibody production and cellular immunity. Each of these cell types are discussed individually.

Granulocytes

Granulopoiesis goes through six maturation stages. Granulocytes are responsible for phagocytosis, chemotaxis, and microbial killing—all essential components of the body's defense system. They also are active in the production of kinins. Kinins increase vascular permeability, cause local vasodilatation, are chemotactic, and may be responsible for margination of granulocytes along walls or small vessels early in inflammation. Granulocytes produce a substance that in the presence of a coagulation factor called the Hageman factor yields active kallikrein, which converts kininogen to bradykinin. In addition, granulocytes are thought to produce pyrogen, the fever producing substance. Most of granulocytic functions take place extravascularly.

After the committed stem cell stage, the line of development is:

- myeloblast
- promyelocyte
- myelocyte
- metamyelocyte
- band form, and
- mature polymorphonuclear granulocyte (Fig. 2-4).

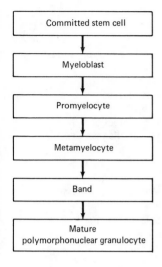

Figure 2-4. Granulocyte development.

The blood granulocyte count is nearly constant in normal subjects. This is achieved by two feedback loops. One loop controls the entrance of the stem cells into the granulopoietic pathway. Stem cells are influenced by a humoral agent known as colony-stimulating activity (CSA), or leukopoietin, thereby influencing this loop. The other loop controls the release of stored mature granulocytes from marrow into the blood. There is evidence that a humoral agent, a neutrophil-releasing factor, may be responsible for this loop.

Granulocytes leave the blood on a random basis, though a few are destroyed when senescent. Although RBCs leave the bloodstream because they die of old age, granulocytes leave the blood because there is a demand for them in the tissues, and the demand does not distinguish between relatively young or old cells. The life span of granulocytes averages about 7 hours.

Granulocytes possess most of the anabolic and catabolic pathways of other body cells, including the following biochemical features:

1. Aerobic glycolysis.
2. Hexose monophosphate shunt pathway.
3. Leukocyte alkaline phosphatase, an enzyme closely linked with neutrophilic granules.
4. Myeloperoxidase, an enzyme that accounts for the green color of pus.
5. Lysozyme (muramidase), an enzyme associated with the lysosomes of granulocytes and monocytes.

Neutrophils
Neutrophils are the most numerous of the granulocytes. They represent 50 to 70 percent of the total number of WBCs. Band neutrophils are a slightly immature form and account for about 3 percent of the total WBC. A "shift to the left" is a term describing an increase in the number of bands and other

TABLE 2-3. WHITE BLOOD CELLS

Type	Percent of WBC	Comments
Neutrophils	50–70	↑ Inflammation Invasive tumors
Eosinophils	2–4	↑ Allergic states Drug reactions Parasitic infections Some skin disease and neoplasms
Basophils	0.5	↑ Asthma Some carcinomas Inflammatory bowel disease Chronic inflammation
Macrophages	5–7	↑ Chronic infections Liver disease Neutropenia
Lymphocytes	20–35	↑ Some carcinomas
Plasma cells	?	↑ Multiple myeloma

less mature neutrophils. It usually occurs with localized infectious processes, for instance, appendicitis. The greater the shift, the more severe the infection. In contrast, a "shift to the right" describes an increase in mature neutrophils. It is associated with pernicious anemia and chronic morphine addiction. In early chronic myelogenous leukemia, one can see both shifts (Table 2–3).

Neutrophils are normally produced in the bone marrow, and after a short time in the blood, move into tissues and body cavities. The only well documented function of the neutrophil is phagocytosis. Neutrophils are capable of effective phagocytosis only when mature. They are attracted to areas of inflammation and bacterial proliferation. The number of neutrophils increases with inflammation, invasive tumors, and myeloproliferative disorders.

The administration of pharmacologic doses of adrenal glucocorticosteroids induces an increase in the number of neutrophils. However, the number of mature effective cells is decreased, which is why clients on steroids are more prone to develop serious infections.

Eosinophils

Eosinophils represent 2 to 4 percent of the total number of leukocytes. They are weakly phagocytic. Their function is thought to be a detoxification of foreign proteins. Their number increases during an allergic attack as they collect at the site of antigen–antibody reactions and remove that complex from the blood after the completion of the immune response. They probably also contribute to fibrin clot digestion by secreting plasmin, an enzyme responsible for clot digestion.

Eosinophils are present in large numbers in the mucosa of the intestinal tract and in lung tissues, thereby protecting the body against foreign proteins. The number of eosinophils increase in drug reactions, such as codeine or penicillin sensitivity; allergic reactions, such as asthma; parasitic infections; skin diseases, such as exfoliative dermatitis; some neoplasms, such as Hodgkin's disease and metastatic cancer of the lung; hypereosinophilic syndromes, such as periarteritis nodosa; and infections, such as tuberculosis and leprosy. Corticosteroids sharply decrease the number of eosinophils.

Basophils

Basophils are not phagocytic. They are similar to the mast cells that are located near many of the body's capillaries and secrete heparin into the bloodstream. Basophils have a high content of heparin and histamine. Basophils are vital for the prevention of clot formation and growth, and accelerating the removal of fat particles from blood after a fatty meal. They play an important role in such systemic allergic reactions as anaphylaxis by undergoing degranulation and liberating heparin and histamine into the bloodstream.

The number of basophils increases during such states as asthma, some carcinomas, inflammatory bowel disease, hypothyroidism, after splenectomy, and during estrogen administration. They remain slightly increased during states of chronic inflammation. Inflammation has a coagulant effect upon the RBCs, and this may be the reason why basophils are increased. They are responding to the body's need for more heparin to prevent the coagulation process from consuming red blood cells.

Monocytes and Macrophages

Monocytes and macrophages are the mobile components of the reticuloendothelial system (RES). Most of the RES is composed of fixed cells lining sinusoids in lymph nodes, liver, and bone marrow. Monocytes are immature cells, released from the bone marrow shortly after their precursors have completed the last mitotic division, and then migrate into tissues or body cavities, to mature into free macrophages or fixed macrophages. Macrophages are present in all tissues, but are especially dense in filter organs such as the liver, spleen, lung, and lymph nodes where they constitute a guard system against invading organisms. This is how they fit into the RES.

Macrophages are very efficient phagocytes for bacteria, extraneous matter, and dead neutrophils. They even have the capacity to engulf whole RBCs and malarial parasites, and are especially efficient in phagocytizing necrotic tissues in chronic inflammation. Free macrophages are wandering cells that migrate from blood through the endothelial membranes of the vascular system to trap material for phagocytosis. They are found at sites of inflammation, and in peritoneal, pleural, and synovial fluid. Fixed macrophages, or histiocytes, phagocytize microorganisms, cellular and noncellular debris. They are in the spleen, lymph nodes, bone marrow, capillaries of the liver, adrenal glands, pituitary, lung, and endothelial cells of all blood vessels. Macrophages, together with lymphocytes, are involved in immune responses that include programming lymphocytes for antibody formation and containment of intracellular parasites, viruses, protozoa, mycobacterium and fungi.

Monocytes have a unique sensitivity to corticosteroids. They show impaired movement, chemotaxis, and bactericidal activity after exposure to low concentrations of hydrocortisone, again displaying the reason why clients on steroids are at increased risk for infection.

The number of monocytes is increased in chronic infections, liver disease, during recovery from infections, and in neuropenia.

Lymphocytes

Lymphocytes represent 20 to 35 percent of the total number of leukocytes. They are leukocytes that originate and differentiate in the primary lymphoid structures of the bone marrow and the thymus gland, and then are distributed to the secondary lymphoid tissues of the lymph nodes, spleen, liver, and intestines.

The precursor of the lymphocyte is thought to be the multipotential stem cell. Development occurs in the following sequence: lymphoblast, prolymphocyte, and mature lymphocyte. The mature lymphocyte differentiates into cells capable of either expressing cell-mediated immune responses or secreting immunoglobulins. The influence for the former type of differentiation is the thymus gland, which leads to a thymus-dependent lymphocyte, or T cell. The site of formation of lymphocytes with potential to differentiate into antibody producing cells has only been identified in chickens, the bursa of Fabricus. Therefore, lymphocytes from the bursa equivalent in humans, probably the bone marrow, are called B cells.

Lymphocytes are discussed in greater detail in the immunity section.

Plasma Cells

Plasma cells are free cells found in lymphatic tissues, lymph nodes, spleen, and connective tissue throughout the body. They are the primary producers of immunoglobins, or antibodies.

There is a close relationship between lymphocytes and plasma cells. After antigenic stimulation, the B lymphocytes have the capacity to differentiate into antibody producing plasma cells. B lymphocytes are actually considered plasma cell precursors. This conversion of B lymphocytes to plasma cells is a highly specific conversion because only those antigens that chemically and physically fit with the already produced immunoglobulin can trigger the reaction. The role of the antigen is very specific. It stimulates the differentiation of the B lymphocyte cell and induces a high level of antibody formation.

Plasma cells can also originate via a maturation pathway. This occurs in the following developmental sequence: stem cell, plasmablast, proplasmacyte, and plasmacytes.

Inflammation and phagocytosis are important, nonspecific defense mechanisms. Much of the work for these two activities is done by the WBCs. Inflammation can be initiated by any cellular injury. It is a sequence of events of WBC activity, vascular responses, and utilizes substances from a number of sources, including the autonomic system and damaged cells. It is an important step, for it helps in the destruction of unwanted agents, prepares for the healing process, and maintains homeostasis.

When tissue injury occurs, large quantities of histamine, bradykinin, serotonin, and other substances are liberated by damaged tissues into the surrounding area. These substances, especially histamine, increase the local blood flow and the permeability of the vascular system, which allows large quantities of fluid and protein, including fibrinogen, into the tissues. This leads to local extracellular edema. The extracellular fluid and the lymphatic fluid clot because of the coagulating effect of tissue exudates on the leaking fibrinogen. This effect walls off the area (Figs. 2–5 through 2–8). The area is quickly invaded by neutrophils and macrophages. A combination of chemical substances released from the inflamed tissues, including a leukocytosis-inducing factor that diffuses from the inflamed tissues into the blood and is carried to the bone marrow. This substance dilates the venous sinusoids of the bone marrow, and causes the release of neutrophils and other WBCs to be immediately transferred from the bone marrow storage pool into the circulating blood. Within a few hours, the number of circulating neutrophils increases by four to five times. The emigration of leukocytes to the area of injury takes place by a process known as diapedesis. Leukocytes cross the vessel walls via interendothelial junctions.

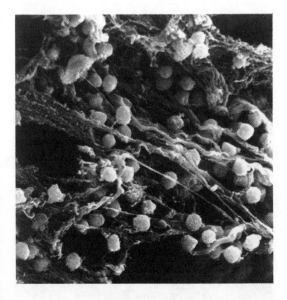

Figure 2–5. Scanning electron micrograph (SEM) showing leukocytes in inflamed tissue. *(From Ryan, G. B., & Majno, G. Inflammation. Kalamazoo, Mich: Upjohn Co., 1977.)*

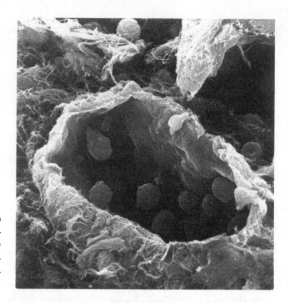

Figure 2-6. Leukocytes stuck to the wall of a venule in an inflamed tissue (SEM). *(From Ryan, G. B., & Majno, G. Inflammation. Kalamazoo, Mich: Upjohn Co., 1977.)*

Macrophages exude into the area about 4 hours after the injury. Their peak phagocytic activity is reached after 16 to 24 hours. They secrete large quantities of lysosomes, which lyse bacterial walls. If the tissue is infected with pyogenic (pus producing) bacteria, the influx of neutrophils is greatly enhanced and sustained.

The signs and symptoms of inflammation—heat, pain, swelling, redness—are the result of kinins, compromised blood flow in the area, histamine release, and other factors.

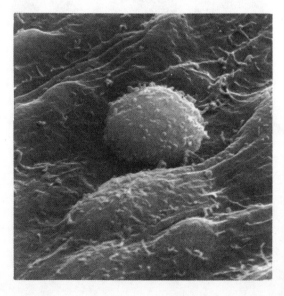

Figure 2-7. A leukocyte stuck to a venular wall and probably preparing to crawl through it (see Figure 2-8) to reach the tissue (SEM). *(From Ryan, G. B., & Majno, G. Inflammation. Kalamazoo, Mich: Upjohn Co., 1977.)*

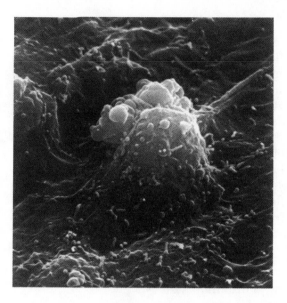

Figure 2-8. A leukocyte crawling through a venular wall (SEM). *(From Ryan, G. B., & Majno, G. Inflammation. Kalamazoo, Mich: Upjohn Co., 1977.)*

The isolation of the inflammatory process can lead to abscess formation, thereby limiting the spread of microorganisms. The abscess is filled with pus, which contains living bacteria, proteolytic enzymes, and dead neutrophils.

Phagocytosis, or cellular eating, may occur prior to or simultaneously with the inflammatory process. Phagocytosis, while not dependent upon, is increased by the inflammatory responses, and is greatly enhanced by the immune response.

Phagocytosis is the process that removes injured cells and antigens from an area, and is performed by neutrophils and macrophages. The formation of an inflammatory exudate. composed primarily of neutrophils, monocytes, and macrophages, occurs rapidly in response to a local infection. This process of tissue damage initiates some form of stimulus that induces the following sequence of events.

Neutrophils primarily phagocytize bacteria, which are then digested by lysosomal enzymes. Macrophages digest large particles, such as debris and foreign materials. The process involves the steps of adhesivity, diapedesis, chemotaxis, opsonization, phagocytosis, and killing. Adhesivity, or margination, is the process whereby phagocytes slow down and adhere to the vessel wall and site of antigen. Diapedesis is the process whereby neutrophils and macrophages can squeeze through pores of small blood vessels. A small portion of the cell slides through the pore at a time. Chemotaxis, the attraction of cells toward chemical substances, is a response to the liberation of serum chemicals called chemotoxins. It is a complex reaction that causes the phagocytes, primarily the neutrophils, to be drawn to the affected area. Some of the chemotoxis are the kinins, bacterial products, certain components of complement, and lysosomal contents. Chemotaxis may also involve the complement system, the blood coagulation system, and interactions between kallikrein and plasminogen activator. An antibody can attach itself to the phagocytes, which causes the offending agent to adhere to the phagocyte so it can be destroyed. This antibody is known as an opsonin. Phagocytosis then takes place. It is the most important function of the neutrophils and macrophages. The ingested organism is then destroyed by lysosomal enzymes. Neutrophils can destroy 5 to 20 bacteria before they are inactivated. Neutrophil phagocytosis is initiated within minutes after antigenic stimulation, and the neutrophil usually dies in the process. Macrophages arrive at the injured area a little later, have a longer life span, and secrete large amounts of lysozyme.

Steroids exert their antiinflammatory effect by stabilizing lysosome membranes and preventing the release of chemotactic substances, and by inhibiting the migration of cells to inflammatory sites.

The WBCs exert a very powerful defense mechanism through phagocytosis and inflammation. Their contributions to immunity are further discussed in a later section.

Thrombocytic Cell System: Thrombopoiesis

Platelets

Platelets, or thrombocytes, are the smallest of the formed elements of the blood. They are cell fragments unique in their ability to adhere to injured blood vessel walls and from cellular aggregates or hemostatic plugs. The platelet is a small fragment of a giant bone marrow precursor cell, called the megakaryocyte. The developmental sequence is thought to be as follows: multipotent stem cell, committed stem cell, megakaryoblast, promegakaryocyte, megakaryocyte, and platelets. Platelet production in the marrow is regulated to meet the requirements for circulating platelets, presumably by a humoral stimulator, known as thrombopoietin. After platelets leave the marrow, they are taken up by the spleen. They equilibrate slowly with the circulating platelet pool. At any moment, 80 percent of platelets are circulating and 20 percent are localized in the spleen. Platelets move freely between these two pools. If the spleen enlarges markedly, up to 80 percent of the platelets may be pooled in the spleen.

Platelets have a life span of 7 to 14 days. About 15 percent of the circulating platelets are continually being consumed in normal intravascular clot formation. The platelet count is normally 150,000 to 300,000 per cu mm.

The level of catecholamines in the blood has an effect on platelet levels. Adrenalin administered clinically produces an immediate 30 to 50 percent increase in the platelet count. This is probably the result of platelet mobilization from the spleen. Exercise also leads to an increase in the platelet count, even in postsplenectomy clients. It is therefore believed that the lung also releases platelets into the circulation. This increase in platelets equilibrates within 30 minutes. Platelets are also increased at high altitudes and with hypoxia.

Platelets perform several important functions:

1. Hemostatic plugs help to stop the flow of blood from damaged blood vessels;
2. Platelets are a source of phospholipids, which are essential in reactions of the coagulation system plasma proteins;
3. Platelets help to maintain the integrity of vascular endothelium by repairing small vascular injuries.

Platelets effect most of their hemostatic function via aggregation and adhesion. Aggregation refers to platelets attaching to one another. Adhesion describes the attachment of platelets to blood vessel walls or foreign surfaces.

Platelet adhesion to subendothelial connection tissue structures, especially collagen, basement membrane, and so on, follows within a moment of any break in the endothelium. Adherent platelets release adenosine diphosphate (ADP), which leads to aggregation of platelets. The aggregated platelets and RBCs form a loose, primary hemostatic plug. Thrombin is generated by the plasma coagulation system, activated by contact with the damaged vessel wall. The platelets respond to the thrombin in a response known as the "release reaction" whereby they release their intracellular constituents into the surrounding plasma, more ADP, ATP, serotonin, catecholamines, potassium, calcium, and platelet factor 4. The platelet plug is now fused into a tightly packed mass referred to as a secondary hemostatic plug. As higher concentrations of thrombin are generated, fibrin strands develop and solidify the plug.

There is a number of limiting reactions that normally prevent massive platelet deposition after small injury. These are continued flow of blood past growing platelet plugs, which removes loosely adherent platelets and dilutes the concentration of ADP and actions of plasma enzymes that degrade ADP.

CHAPTER 3
Immunity

Since ancient times, observant individuals have noted that a person recovering from a certain infectious disease becomes resistant to reinfection by that same disease. From these observations have come the fundamental concepts underlying the complex and ever-evolving field of immunobiology.

Immunity is a defense. It is the essential function by which vertebrates maintain their functional integrity when threatened by the entry of foreign chemical substances into the body. It is a series of events that protect the body against foreign agents. Immunity implies the capacity to distinguish foreign agents from body constituents, a phenomenon known as self-tolerance.

Whenever the body recognizes the presence of an invading organism or a protein material that it cannot identify as a part of itself, the body protects itself through the immune response. Normally, the immune system responds to an invasion of foreign substances or antigens, by producing immune response components, antibodies and sensitized lymphocytes. In an immune system damaged by pathologic changes, however, an immune response may occur in response to some of the body's own proteins, resulting in the production of autoantibodies. These pathologic conditions in which the body directs the immune response against itself are called autoimmune diseases.

Our immune system recognizes most proteins, bacteria, viruses, and parasites that are not part of the normal body environment as foreign and will initiate an immune response. Those substances capable of eliciting an immune response are called antigens or immunogens. An antigen is a substance that, due to its chemical configuration, is capable of reacting with an antibody. An immunogen is any substance that induces a detectable immune response (humoral, cellular, or both) when introduced into a host.

Specifically, antigens are chemical substances that are nearly always protein in nature and are viewed by the body as an attacking force. The structures of antigenic microorganisms, e.g., bacteria and viruses, are protein as are almost all the toxins that they manufacture and release. Microorganisms and their toxins are termed antigenic because they stimulate the immune response. To be an antigen, a substance must have a high molecular weight.

TABLE 3-1. NATURAL (NONSPECIFIC) IMMUNE DEFENSES

Inflammation
Phagocytosis
Genetic susceptibility
Pyrogen and body temperature
Age
Interferon
Natural antibodies
Body pH
Epithelial surfaces

There are substances of low molecular weight called haptens against which the body can develop immunity under certain conditions. Haptens include drugs, chemical constituents in dust, and breakdown products of animal dander. To stimulate an immune response, a hapten must first combine with an antigenic substance. Together, the hapten and antigen stimulate the body to produce antibodies and sensitized lymphocytes against themselves, which results in their destruction. As a result, if the individual is exposed for a second time to either the antigen or the hapten, the immune response is elicited.

Antibodies are proteins secreted by plasma cells in response to a specific antigen. The antigen–antibody complex consists of an antibody linked to a specific antigen. An antibody is known as an immunoglobulin or Ig. There are five classes of immunoglobulins IgG, IgA, IgM, IgE, and IgD. They are either natural or acquired. Natural antibodies, usually IgM, are normally present without previous contact with the antigen against which it is directed. Acquired antibodies arise as part of the humoral response.

The immune system is composed of natural and acquired defenses (Table 3–1). Natural defenses are nonspecific. They are present from birth or may develop throughout life. They include anatomical and chemical barriers and processes. They exist without apparent prior contact with an immunogen and include the following: inflammation; phagocytosis; genetic susceptibility; pyrogen, body temperature; age; interferon; natural antibodies; body PH; and epithelial surfaces.

Acquired defenses go into operation when natural defenses fail and allow a foreign organism into the body. It enables the body to protect itself against foreign organisms and protein substances for which it does not have a natural immunity.

NATURAL NONSPECIFIC DEFENSE MECHANISMS

Nonspecific defenses are discussed first as they represent the initial protection mechanism.

The intact skin acts as the first line of defense against bacterial invasion. Epithelial surfaces are present on the skin and its appendages—respiratory, gastrointestinal, and genitourinary mucosa. Epithelial cells have receptors for attachment of certain antigens, which are important in maintaining the normal body flora. Secretory IgA is an antibody linked to epithelial cells, secreted by skin, gastrointestinal, and genitourinary mucosa, and prevents pathogens from attaching to epithelial cells. This is obviously an important function because all of the potential entry sites to the body are epithelial in nature, and are therefore protected. Secretory IgA enhances the natural defense system of the body by offering protection against the effects of proteolytic enzymes in bacteria. Epithelial surfaces are an effective barrier against microorganisms because of their structure and pH, and because they continually exfoliate. In addition, there is some local production of chemical antimicrobial and antiviral agents. Both bacterial attachment to epithelial receptors and secretory IgA prevent attachment of pathogenic organisms.

Pyrogen, produced primarily by granulocytes, is a class of substances that cause an increase in body temperature. This may have an inhibitory effect on bacteria.

Interferon is a glycoprotein produced by any cell to protect the body against viral infections. It acts by preventing viral reproduction in the cells. Interferon production can be stimulated by virus, bacterial endotoxins, and other substances. Interferon is capable of inhibiting division of both normal and malignant cells; it enhances macrophage activity and stimulates cytotoxic T lymphocyte function. Therefore, interferon is being used experimentally in a number of clinical situations.

Other nonspecific defenses include body pH, age, and natural antibodies. The pH of the blood and the body fluids is maintained within a very narrow range. Microorganisms do not thrive at this pH and therefore, their growth is inhibited. The sera of humans contains natural antibodies which, in low titer, are bactericidal. In the presence of complement, these antibodies are frequently bacteriolytic toward a number of gram-negative bacterial species. The absence of such antibodies in the serum of germ-free animals suggest that they originate in response to food and microbial antigens absorbed from the bowel.

The fetus receives a library of preformed antibody from its mother, reflecting most of her experiences with infectious agents. Because the immunoglobulins are passively transferred, they have a finite half life of beween 20 and 30 days and concentration in serum falls rapidly within the first few months of life, reaching the lowest levels between the second and fourth month. This period is known as physiologic hypogammaglobulinemia. During the course of the first few years, the levels of antibody increases because of the exposure of the maturing infant to antigens in the environment.

ACQUIRED HOST DEFENSES

The acquired, or specific, host defenses include a number of mechanisms that are stirred into action when nonspecific defenses fail (Table 3–2). They re-

TABLE 3-2. ACQUIRED (SPECIFIC) DEFENSES

1. The mononuclear phagocyte system (reticuloendothelial system) and lymphatic system
2. Biological self
3. Humoral immunity
4. Cellular immunity
5. Complement system
6. Tissue signatures

quire immunological life experience before they can be activated. We are born with these specific defenses but we must be exposed to various antigens before they can begin to work. These defenses include: reticuloendothelial system and lymphatic system (mononuclear phagocyte system), biological self, humoral immunity, cellular immunity, complement system, and tissue signatures.

Specific immunity is that portion of the immune system that recognizes antigens as nonself and is capable of more precise immunological reactions than the nonspecific arm of the immune system. Here, the immunological response is unique and tailored to each antigen.

The *mononuclear phagocyte system*, also known as reticuloendothelial system (RES), includes all the cells and structures that recognize, respond to, and remember antigens. Functionally, these cells are remarkable for their ability to phagocytize particulate matter, and for their significant roles in humoral defense and metabolism. Included within this system are:

1. Primary and secondary lymphoid tissue.
2. Lymphatic cells, T and B cells.
3. A network of phagocytic cells, macrophages, within lymphatic and other organs.

Lymphoid tissue is composed of two groups: central lymphoid tissue (or primary) and secondary lymphoid tissue. Central lymphoid tissues include thymus, bone marrow, spleen, and liver. These are structures that are essential for stimulating the development and differentiation of the primitive lymphocyte into mature T or B cells. Secondary lymphoid tissues include the lymphatic system and the spleen. The immune response usually occurs initially within the secondary lymphoid tissues, which have specific areas populated by T or B cells.

The lymphatic system consists of lymphatic capillaries, ducts, and lymph nodes. The lymphatic capillaries are an intricate network of distensible vessels that collect lymph. Their main function is drainage. They coalesce into progressively larger vessels until they finally form the two main channels: the thoracic (or left lymphatic duct) and the right lymphatic duct. The thoracic duct drains the lower part of the body, the left side of the head, arm, and chest. The right lymphatic duct empties the right side of the head, arm, and chest. Both ducts drain into the internal jugulars and subclavian veins.

Lymph, a watery interstitial fluid, has the same composition as the tissue fluid from where it is draining. It contains antibodies, lymphocytes, granulocytes, and enzymes.

Lymph nodes are bean-shaped bodies occurring at frequent intervals, usually in chains, along lymphatic vessels. They remove foreign particles from the blood. All lymph passes through at least one node and is rid of bacteria, dead cells, and other foreign particles and debris. In the node, T cells and B cells have specific locations, the B cells in the cortex and medulla and the T cells in the paracortical areas. The nodes serve as centers for proliferation of lymphocytes and other immunocompetent cells, this process being stimulated by antigens.

BIOLOGICAL SELF

Native proteins are recognized as "self" by the immune system of the body. Self is anything synthesized according to the individual's particular genetic code. Nonself, or antigens, is produced by a different set of chromosomes and evokes the immune response.

The RES recognizes substances that are different from self and can evoke the immune response. Self-molecules do not ordinarily produce immune reactions because of a natural tolerance developed during fetal life. This tolerance is probably secondary to the inactivation of certain clones, or groups of cells from a single parent cells, in fetal life. The recognition of self is a phenomenon known as biological self and is considered part of specific immunity.

The immune response can be elicited by:

1. Transplanted cells.
2. Microorganisms.
3. Native material altered by a genetic mutation or by physical structural change.
4. A foreign molecule that becomes attached to a native protein and produces an antigen.
5. Native material located in an abnormal location.

Autoimmune diseases are those in which structural or functional changes are produced by immunologically competent cells or antibodies against normal components of the body. Previously native proteins are not recognized as such for a multitude of reasons, and the immune system produces antibodies in reaction to the presence of nonself proteins. Autoimmunity, in contrast, is defined as immunological reactivity against self-antigens. It reflects a loss of tolerance, and activation of immune cells that are normally unresponsive. Frequently we lose some of our immune tolerance as we grow older, as a result of destruction of some of the body's tissues which then release considerable quantities of antigen. These antigens circulate in the body and lead to sensitized lymphocyte and antibody formation. The antigens can also combine with other proteins, from bacteria or viruses for instance, and create a new antigen that can then cause immunological reactions. The resulting sensitized lymphocytes and antibodies attack the body's tissues.

The phenomenon of autoimmunity is much more prevalent than the autoimmune diseases, and is mediated by autoantibodies. An autoantibody is a specific immunoglobulin that reacts with certain serum proteins and other cellular components. About 50 percent of people in their sixth and seventh decades have at least one autoantibody without any signs of clinical disease.

Aberrations in the immune defense system are believed to play an important role in the pathogenesis of rheumatoid arthritis, systemic lupus erythematosus, and a number of other connective tissue diseases. In these diseases, there is a breakdown in the normal antigen recognition system such that antibodies react with antigens present in the host's own tissues or there is an immune response that is mediated by T cells.

IMMUNITY

After exposure to an antigen, an immune response confers immunity against that antigen. Antibodies and sensitized cells are produced that have the ability to recognize, react with, and kill that antigen. Specific responses take two forms that usually develop in parallel, humoral immunity via B lymphocytes, and cell-mediated or cellular immunity via T lymphocytes.

A great deal of immunity is acquired in childhood. By the time a child is 6 years old, he has a mature immune system. This occurs through the build up of memory cells, or immunological memory. The first time a person encounters an antigen, he must undergo a primary response. If the antigen is bacterial, for instance, the humoral immune system is stimulated into action. First, the antigen is processed by a macrophage. This processing is an important step whereby the antigen is made to be much more toxic to the body than it would be on its own, thereby prompting the immune system into action. After the macrophage processing step, the B lymphocyte proliferates and forms a clone, or a group of cells that are exactly identical. Each B lymphocyte within that clone is specific to this particular antigen. From that clone emerges the plasma cell, which is also specific to this particular antigen. The plasma cell produces the antibody and again, it is specific to the particular antigen. Memory cells are produced simultaneously.

On the other hand, if the antigen is viral, the cellular arm of the immune system is stimulated into action and undergoes a very similar process. The viruses are processed by the macrophage. From there, a clone of T lymphocyte develops, specific to the particular antigen. From the clone emerges sensitized T lymphocytes, all specific to the particular antigen, and memory cells.

These steps constitute the primary immune response. The initial encounter with an antigen stimulates the primary immune response and requires 4 to

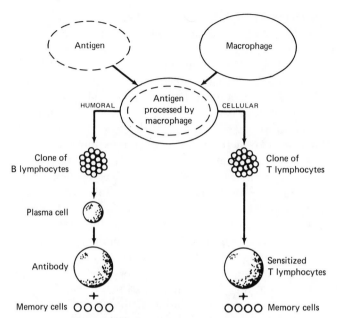

Figure 3-1. Primary immune response.

10 days before it is complete. This length of time is the reason why children become sick more often than do adults; they are encountering many new antigens and are building up a mature immune system, complete with innumerable memory cells against all sorts of antigens.

The second and subsequent encounters with antigens stimulate the secondary response which, because of the presence of memory cells, is faster, stronger, and more persistent than the primary response (Fig. 3–1).

Humoral Immunity

Humoral immunity is initiated by B lymphocytes. The term humoral means that it is an immunity transferrable by serum. B cells are lymphocytes derived from bone marrow stem cells and are dependent for their maturation and development on a lymphoepithelial organ, the equivalent of the chick's bursa of Fabricus. In humans, the bursa's equivalent is probably the bone marrow. After transformation of the stem cell to a B lymphocyte, usually a few months after birth, they migrate to lymphoid tissues where they further differentiate.

Humoral immunity involves two systems: the antibody and the complement systems.

B lymphocytes are precursors of the antibody secreting cell, the plasma cell. Antibodies are released from the highly differentiated plasma cell. Plasma cells are formed when groups of antigen specific B lymphocytes, or clones, respond to the presence of antigen. This antigen specificity is determined by a receptor site on the B lymphocyte cell membrane. Each plasma cell produces only one type of antibody. Other activated B cells remain quiescent and turn into memory cells.

The presentation of the antigen to the B cell is a complex process that involves macrophages and usually a helper T cell. The macrophage presents the antigen to the B cell in a form that it can respond to, and the T cell gives a signal to the B cell that is necessary for the production of antigen. When an antigen is initially exposed to serum, little or no antibody can be detected for a period of time. During this delay, antigen is recognized by B lymphocytes. The B cell divides and differentiates into a plasma cell to form antibody specific to that antigen. This primary antibody response is equivalent 4 to 10 days after initial exposure to the antigen. The first type of antibody formed is IgM. As the immune response continues, it matures and ultimately produces IgG.

The antibody usually does not reach high levels or persist unless a second encounter with the antigen occurs. When a secondary antibody response occurs, an antibody is produced within 1 to 2 days and the antibody titer may be up to 50 times that in the primary response. The second response maintains antibody titers at high levels and falls slowly over a period of months. Therefore the secondary response is faster, stronger, and more persistent than the primary response with antibody levels being boosted to even higher levels with each exposure to an antigen.

Subsequent to the primary response, the immune system retains a memory of the antigen via B lymphocyte memory cells. Even after prolonged intervals, an individual can respond, through the secondary response, by means of rapid mobilization of antibody forming cells. IgG is the primary antibody in the secondary response, although some IgM is also present (Table 3–3).

TABLE 3–3. IMMUNOGLOBULINS

Class	Percent of Total	Activity
IgG	75	Active against most bacteria, some parasites, viruses, and fungi Fixes complement Primary antibody of the primary immune response Crosses placenta
IgA	15	Present in most body secretions Activates complement through alternate properdin pathway
IgM	10	Fixes complement Efficient agglutination against particulate antigens (RBC, bacteria) - transfusion, reactions Common antibody to blood group substances
IgE	0.002	Allergic reactions
IgD	1	Unknown ? membrane receptor on lymphocytes

The antigen–antibody reaction results in the death of the antigen through one or more of the following steps.

1. Precipitation—insoluble antibody, in combination with soluble antigen, leads to precipitation of the antigen–antibody complex. This leads to formation of a clump that is quickly destroyed by phagocytes.
2. Agglutination—when an antigen attaches itself to particulate matter, for instance a red blood cell, the antigen–antibody complex forms clumps. This happens in transfusion reactions.
3. Neutralization—at times, an antibody can neutralize bacterial toxins.
4. Opsonization—a reaction between antigen and antibody that cause the antigen to become sticky and makes it easier for phagocytes to engulf them.

Complement fixation describes a series of enzymatic reactions resulting in antigen destruction by lysis. Complement is an encompassing term for 11 serum proteins circulating in inactive form. They comprise 10 to 15 percent of the serum globulins. They have a nonspecific function in immune and nonimmune reactions. They can function as a defense by promoting removal of infectious agents, or as a threat by triggering destructive reactions in host tissue.

Complement lyses cells by fixing to any cell with IgM or IgG attached to it. The immunoglobulin guides the complement to specific targets, which spares other cells. Complement is present in serum in inactive form until fixed, or activated, by an antibody in what is known as the classical pathway. This pathway is a series of events in which a specific antibody, IgG or IgM, identifies and coats an antigen; a complement protein recognizes and binds with the antibody; a series of enzymatic reaction is activated that involves all the complement proteins, resulting in cell lysis. This is complement fixation. The antigen is coated with immunoglobulin (usually IgG or IgM). The complement proteins recognize this coated cell as a red flag, and go in and destroy any cell to which these immunoglobulins are attached. There is also an alternate, or properdin, pathway whereby substances other than antigen–antibody complexes, such as bacterial endotoxins and aggregated immunoglobulins, react with properdin, a serum factor, producing an enzyme that activates the pathway. This alternate pathway is especially important in the body's defense against gastrointestinal (GI) tract bacteria.

Despite the fact that there are 11 proteins encompassed by the term complement, only nine have been numerically designated, C1 through C9, with C1 having three subcomponents, C1q, C1r, and C1s. C1 is primarily synthesized by intestinal epithelium, C2 and C4 produced by macrophages, C3, C6, and C9 by the liver, and C5 and C8 by the spleen.

The complement system proteins cause cell lysis through one or more of the following steps:

1. Agglutination—complement enzymes change the surface of some of the antigenic agents so they adhere to each other, form clumps and are destroyed by phagocytes.
2. Neutralization—complement enzymes can neutralize viruses.
3. Opsonization and phagocytosis—complement proteins and their proteolytic enzymes alter the antigen's cell membrane and make it vulnerable to phagocytosis and lysis.
4. Chemotaxis—complement products attract killer T cells and macrophages to dispatch and devour the antibody coated invader.
5. Lysis—proteolytic enzymes of the complement system digest portions of the cell membrane, leading to its rupture. Destruction of the alien cell results in pus, which is the remains of cells, macrophages, killer T cells, complement, antibodies, and so on.
6. Inflammatory effects—complement products elicit a local inflammatory reaction leading to hyperemia, coagulation of proteins in tissues, and other aspects of the inflammatory process.

The complement response hinges on the body's recognition of self. As long as the immunoglobulins attach themselves to antigens, the complement system is a very efficient process. If the cell attacked by the complement represents a threat, this immune reaction can protect life. However, if the body recognizes self as foreign, as it happens in donor organs, the complement system mechanisms can result in catastrophic consequences. Some other examples of complement disorders include systemic lupus erythematosus, hereditary angioedema, glomerulonephritis, and graft versus host disease.

Cellular Immunity

Cellular immunity is a function of the T lymphocyte. In contrast to humoral immunity, cellular immunity cannot be transferred from one individual to another by plasma. It is dependent on the presence of immune cells. Some major functions of cellular immunity include:

1. Protection against most viruses and fungi.
2. Mediation of cutaneous delayed hypersensitivity reactions, such as the purified protein derivative (PPD) test.
3. Rejection of transplanted organs.
4. Response to slowly developing bacterial diseases such as tuberculosis.
5. Immunological surveillance against cancer cells.
6. As helper or suppressor cells to modulate the overall immune response to a specific challenge.

The T lymphocyte originates in the bone marrow, and migrates to the thymus where it is acted upon by thymic hormones. The cell then moves to the lymphoid tissue, where it differentiates into clones of antigen specific T cells.

TABLE 3-4. T LYMPHOCYTES

Subset	Function
Killer T cells	Produce lymphokines
	Kill cells
Helper T cells	Produce lymphokines
	Participate in antibody production
Suppressor T cells	Modulate the overall immune system
Memory T cells	Immunologic memory

There are four subsets of T cells that participate in many phases of the immune response (Table 3-4).

1. Killer T cells or cytotoxic T cells—they react directly with target cells and kill them and/or they produce lymphokines, a cell killing agent. Killer T cells arise from the proliferation of selected antigen specific T cells once an antigen has been processsed. They are also known as effector or T cells.
2. Helper T cells—they help B cells in bringing about antibody production. They also produce lymphokines.
3. Suppressor T cells—they diminish B cell and possibly T cell activity, thereby modulating the overall immune system. They prevent the cellular or humoral arms of the immune system from overpowering the other.
4. Memory T cells—they respond to challenges by antigens previously encountered by the RES.

The T lymphocyte recognizes a foreign antigen on the surface of macrophages and responds by binding to it, enlarging and proliferating into a clone of sensitized T cells that migrate to the antigen site. The antigen is destroyed by direct participation of the killer T cell as well as by lymphokine secretion. Lymphokines have many different functions and act on different kinds of cells including macrophages, lymphocytes, neutrophils, eosinophils, and tissue cells (Table 3-5).

TABLE 3-5. LYMPHOKINES

Lymphokines	Action
Transfer factor	Affects lymphocytes
	Induces delayed type hypersensitivity
Lymphotoxin	Destroys antigen
Mitogenic factor	Initiates cell division in lymphocytes
Skin reactive factor	Local inflammation
Migration inhibitory factor	Inhibits macrophage migration
Macrophage activation factor	Enhances macrophage functioning
Chemotoxic factor	Pulls macrophages and granulocytes to site of immune response
Interferon	Inhibition of viruses

Interaction

Humoral and cellular immunity are interdependent processes. T and B lymphocyte interactions occur. The complement system serves to bridge cellular and humoral immunity. After the system has been activated by IgG or IgM, one by-product of the complement reaction serves as a chemotactic factor, summoning T lymphocytes and macrophages to the site.

Another area of interaction between the two systems is in the production of antibody. T lymphocytes are not required in the production of antibody, but optimal antibody production occurs after an interaction between T and B lymphocytes. An important difference between cellular and humoral immunity is persistence. Humoral antibodies rarely persist for a few months or at most a few years. Sensitized T lymphocytes have indefinite life spans and persist until they come in contact with their specific antigen.

Macrophages, T lymphocytes, and B lymphocytes cooperate to control the immune response. Usually antigens evoke the reaction of both T and B cells. In any specific instance, however, either humoral or cellular destruction predominates as determined by the antigenic receptors on the cell. In addition to the production of antibody forming plasma cells and cytotoxic T cells, longer lived T and B memory lymphocytes are produced in response to antigens.

In summary, cooperation among T cells, B cells, and macrophages controls the immune response. The process begins with nonspecific phagocytosis, processing, and activation of nonself antigens by macrophages. Antigens processed in this manner are changed for recognition as foreign by the lymphocyte populations.

TISSUE SIGNATURES

There are three systems that describe the most important antigens on red blood cells (RBC), tissues, and other cells. These are the ABO system, the Rh system, and the human lymphocyte antigen (HLA) system.

The ABO system, or blood groups, is concerned with antigens on RBCs designated A and B. They are detected and defined by reactions with specific antibodies. The presence or absence of these antigens is under genetic control (Table 3–6).

The normal adult's plasma contains autoantibodies to the antigens not present on his or her RBCs. Some individuals possess the A antigenic determinant and are of the A blood group; others contained the B determinant and belong to the B blood group. Individuals with blood group O possess neither of these determinants, but contain a heterogenetic, or H antigen.

All mature individuals possess antibodies in their serum, the so-called naturally occurring isoantibodies (isoagglutinins) directed against the antigenic determinant absent from their own erythrocytes. The presence of natural antibodies do not require previous immunization episodes for production. A and

TABLE 3-6. ABO SYSTEM

Blood Type	Percent in Population	Genotype	Antibodies
A	41	AA and AO	A antigen on RBC Anti-B antibodies
B	9	BB and BO	B antigen on RBC Anti-A antibodies
AB	3	AB	A and B antigens on RBC No antibodies "Universal recipient"
O	47	OO	No RBC antigens Both Anti-A and Anti-B antibodies

B antigenic determinants are widespread in nature, and this fact, along with diet and bacterial flora of the gut, providing a continual exposure to these antigens, explains the presence of natural antibodies. Individuals of group A possess anti-B; individuals belonging to group B possess anti-A; and those belonging to group O have both anti-A and anti-B. People with group AB have both antigenic determinants present on their RBCs, one of paternal and the other of maternal origins, and have neither anti-A or anti-B isoagglutinins.

The Rh system is a series of six common types of Rh antigens, each of which is called an Rh factor. Because of the manner of inheritance of these factors, each person will have one of each of three pairs of antigens. Only C, D, and E are antigenic enough to cause significant development of anti-Rh antibodies that are capable of causing transfusion reactions. Anyone who has any of these three antigens is Rh + ; a person without C, D, or E, but with c, d, or e is Rh − . Eighty-five percent of Americans have Rh + blood.

The difference between this system and the ABO system is that spontaneous agglutinins almost never occur. Rh antibodies do not occur naturally. Instead, a person must first be massively exposed to an Rh antigen, usually by a transfusion of blood, or pregnancy, before enough agglutinins develop to cause a significant reaction. When RBCs containing one or more Rh + factors are injected into an Rh − person, anti-Rh agglutinins develop slowly, and peak about 2 to 4 months later. On multiple exposure to the Rh factor, the Rh − person becomes strongly sensitized to the Rh factor and develops a very high titer of anti-Rh agglutinins.

If an Rh − person has never been exposed, a transfusion of Rh + blood causes no reaction. But in some persons, anti-Rh antibodies develop during the next 2 to 4 weeks to cause agglutination of transfused cells that are still circulating in the blood. These cells are hemolyzed by the RES. Thus, a delayed transfusion reaction occurs, though usually mild. On subsequent transfusion of Rh + blood into the same person, who is now immunized against Rh factor, transfusion reaction will be greatly enhanced, and can be as severe as those occurring with types A and B blood. Severe hemolytic disease of the newborn is most commonly caused by Rh incompatibility. Antibody formation in the mother can occur through prior transfusion of incompatible cells, or more commonly as a consequence of previous pregnancies. Seventy-one percent of randomly selected postpartum women have fetal red cells in their blood. Maternal production of antibody to these cells is dependent upon genetic constitution, the number of immunizing cells, and the type of red cell antigen transferred. In general, in the case of Rh incompatibility, the severity of the disease is directly proportional to the number of affected pregnancies.

The major histocompatibility system of humans, the human leukocyte antigen (HLA) system, refers to a group of antigenic substances found on many cell types including white blood cells and platelets. The HLA gene complex is located on the short arm of chromosome 6. At least five closely linked but distinct genes (loci) are known (A, B, C, D, and DR), each of which has many different alleles. The particular combination of alleles at each locus on the same chromosome is called the haplotype; two haplotypes, one from each parent, constitute the genotype. Genetic makeup of HLA is quite complex compared to RBC antigen systems. Each individual may have as many as four of the major antigens. Furthermore, the number of different antigens that exist in the population is large. Over 20 antigens have been identified at each major locus and many of them are fairly common. So, literally thousands of combinations for the four antigen composition are possible in an individual, which is called the HLA type.

The HLA antigens are detected serologically by means of cytotoxicity assays, using peripheral blood lymphocytes as targets. Although HLA-A, B, and C antigens are found on all nucleated cells (except RBC), HLA-D and DR antigens exist only on B lymphocytes, moncytes, epidermal, and endothelial cells.

The HLA system achieved even more significance when it was discovered that certain antigens occurred more frequently in individuals with certain diseases, for instance ankylosing spondylitis, multiple sclerosis, and systemic lupus erythematosus. There is much research being done in this area, and it is clear that some relationship does exist between a particular genetic makeup and the development of certain autoimmune diseases.

CHAPTER 4
Hemostasis

Hemostasis is the process whereby vascular breaks are rapidly repaired, while maintaining fluidity of blood. It involves the interaction of platelets, blood vessels, the coagulation system, and fibrinolytic mechanisms.

Hemostatis is discussed in two parts: extrinsic factors and the coagulation system. Extrinsic factors include vascular and cellular, or platelet mechanisms of hemostasis. The coagulation system involves a cascade reaction of various enzymes that evolve into clot formation.

EXTRINSIC FACTORS IN COAGULATION

Vascular Mechanisms of Hemostasis

Blood normally flows within a continuous lining of overlapping endothelial cells. These endothelial cells are tightly attached to capillary walls, across which the blood's function of metabolic exchange occurs. Larger vessels consist of three components. The intima is the inner surface, which includes the endothelium and the subendothelium, basement membrane, elastic tissue, and collagen fibers. The middle layer is composed of smooth muscle cells, collagen fibers, and occasionally fibroblasts. The outer layer is the adventitia, consisting of fibroblasts, collagen fibers, extracellular connective tissue, small blood vessels, eymphatics, and occasionally nerves.

Endothelial cells modulate thrombosis and vascular permeability because of their position as the interfacing cell between the vessel lumen and the blood. The physiology of the endothelial cell has been receiving intense scrutiny. A primary endothelial function is selective vessel permeability, screening out significant quantities of blood-borne materials. They also appear to be the sites of synthesis of prostaglandins, factor VIII antigen, a basement membranelike material resembling collagen, and fibronectin. These cells contain a complex system of plasminogen activation that may protect against fibrin formation.

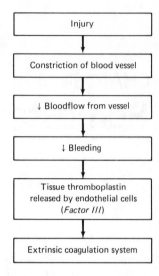

Figure 4-1. Vascular response to injury: Stage I.

They can also process a number of vasoactive materials such as bradykinin, serotonin, and norepinephrine, and appear to possess unique immunological characteristics, having ABO, factor VIII, alpha macroglobulin, and a thromboplastin antigen. This wide variety of antigens found on the endothelial surface may explain its susceptibility to immunological injury. A frequently overlooked function of endothelial cells is phagocytosis, but this may occur only under extreme conditions. The smooth muscle cell is responsible for the synthesis of elastin, collagen, and other connective tissue elements.

The hemostatic response to a torn or ruptured blood vessel must be rapid, localized, and precisely controlled. Specifically, this mechanism must become operational immediately after injury; clot size must be appropriate to the size of the vessel tear and clotting must not occur at any other time.

Vascular damage directly activates all components of the hemostatic response. Immediately after a blood vessel is cut, the wall of the vessel constricts, due to nervous reflexes and local myogenic spasm. This results in a decreased flow of blood from that vessel and reduces the release tissue thromboplastin into inactive form. Tissue thromboplastin, or factor III, is activated by unknown mechanisms and initiates the extrinsic coagulation system. Endothelial cells also synthesize and secrete plasminogen activator and this function may be important in preventing venous thrombosis (Fig. 4–1).

Cellular Mechanisms of Hemostasis

Cellular mechanisms of hemostasis include the activities of the platelets. Platelets can adhere to injured blood vessel walls and form cellular aggregates or hemostatic plugs. These plugs help stop the flow of blood from damaged blood vessels. Platelets are also a source of phospholipids that are essential in

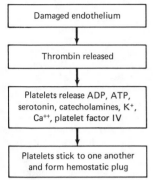

Figure 4-2. Platelet activity in hemostasis: Stage II.

reactions of the coagulation system plasma proteins. They also help to maintain the integrity of the vascular endothelium by repairing small vascular injuries. Phospholipids are procoagulants or substances that tend to favor the occurrence of coagulation. The platelet retains its disc shape until it encounters damaged epithelium. Thrombin is generated by the plasma coagulation system, activated by contact with the damaged vessel wall. The platelets respond to the thrombin in a release reaction by releasing their intracellular constituents into the surrounding plasma—ADP, ATP, serotonin, catecholamines, potassium, calcium, and platelet factor IV. This leads to the adherence of platelets to exposed subendothelial collagen and causes adjacent platelets to stick to the initial platelet layer and each other. This is aggregation. The aggregated platelets and RBCs form a loose, primary hemostatic plug. This is stage 2 of the normal hemostatic response (Fig. 4–2). Thus, there is a positive feedback loop with thrombin causing further release of ADP from platelets.

Endothelial cells relate also to the platelet function. They synthesize von Willebrand protein, which is necessary for normal platelet function in vivo. They synthesize prostacyclin, a powerful inhibitor of platelet aggregation. Because prostacyclin is derived from arachidonic acid via cyclic endoperoxide, aspirin, which inhibits endoperoxide generation, also inhibits prostacyclin formation.

THE COAGULATION SYSTEM

The normal process of hemostasis begins when vascular endothelium is damaged. Platelets are aggregated and form a clot or a platelet fibrin network that is an effective barrier against further escape of blood and a scaffold for the repair of vessel damage.

The next stage of the normal hemostatic response is the formation of a fibrin clot. This occurs via a process of enzymatic reactions involving several plasma proteins, lipids, and ions that transform circulating blood into an insoluble gel through the conversion of soluble fibrinogen to insoluble fibrin.

TABLE 4-1. COAGULATION FACTORS

Factor	Action	Comment
I Fibrinogen	200–400 mg. Synthesized by liver, converted into fibrin by Thrombin Essential for normal platelet function and wound healing	↑ Cirrhosis, nephrosis, myeloma, stress, inflammation, tissue necrosis, pregnancy, oral contraceptives ↓ Hypothyroidism, circulating tissue thromboplastin, liver disease
II Prothrombin	100 mg. Synthesized by liver. Inactive precursor of thrombin. Vitamin K dependent*	↑ Stress, fever, infection, gram negative bacterial endotoxin ↓ Liver disease, vitamin K deficiency, coumorin
III Tissue Thromboplastin	Interacts with factor VII in extrinsic system, arises from virtually any body tissue but especially brain, lungs, prostate, placenta	↓ Liver disease
IV Calcium	9–11 mg, 50% ionized. Only very small quantities of Ca^{++} required for coagulation. Ca^{++} deficiency as cause of coagulopathy rare	Massive blood transfusions with citrated blood products → Hypocalcemia as result of combination of ionized Ca^{++} with EDTA Irreversible reaction which makes Ca^{++} unavailable. Hypergammaglobulinemia also results in abnormal binding of Ca^{++}
V Labile factor, proaccelerin	75–125 mg. Synthesized by liver. Totally consumed in process of coagulation. Essential in formation of prothrombin in final common pathway	↓ Acquired V deficiency—severe liver disease, circulating anticoagulants ↑ Fibrinolysis, pregnancy, oral contraceptives, inflammation
VII Proconvertin, stable factor	72–125 mg. Synthesized in liver. Vitamin K dependent, active only in presence of factor III	↓ Liver disease
VIII Antihemophilic factor	75–150 mg. Primarily synthesized in liver and endothelial cells. Spleen major	Deficiency—classic hemophilia ↑ Inflammation, preg-

TABLE 4-1 (Cont.)

Factor	Action	Comment
	storage site. Required for thromboplastin generation. Procoagulant. Antisera properties. Portion which normally reacts with a specific reactor site on platelets—von Willebrand's factor	nancy, oral contraceptives, after exercise, stress, epinephrine infusions
IX Plasma thromboplastin, Christmas factor	75–150 mg. Vitamin K dependent. Essential role in intrinsic pathway	↓ Coumarin, Christmas disease
X Stuart-Power factor	75–125 mg. Vitamin K dependent. Synthesized in liver. Required for intrinsic thromboplastin formation and for prothrombin conversion. Factor X forms final common pathway	↓ Liver disease, Vitamin K deficiency ↑ Oral contraceptives, pregnancy
XI Plasma thromboplastin antecedent, antihemophilic factor C	70–130 mg. Synthesized in liver, essential in intrinsic pathway	↓ Hemophilia C, liver disease
XII Hageman Factor	70–130 mg. Synthesized in liver. Maintained in inactive form by action of coagulation inhibitors. Reacts with factor XI to form active prothromboplastic substance initiating intrinsic pathway. May serve as a trigger mechanism that translates injury to diverse processes associated with hemostasis and fibrinolysis, humoral and cellular defense, and inflammation	↓ Does not result in hemorrhagic state but a prolonged venous clotting time and PTT
XIII Fibrin stabilizing factor	9–4 u (units). 50% associated associated with platelets, may be derived from platelets	↑ Pregnancy, oral contraceptives, inflammation
	Acts in common pathway of coagulation where it forms a stabilizing bond within fibrin strands	Hereditary deficiency associated with abnormal scar formation and wound dehiscence

*Vitamin K dependent—hepatocyte requires presence of vitamin K for synthesis of these factors. Vitamin K is not stored in the body but is synthesized by bacteria of intestinal flora. Should this flora be disturbed, especially by use of certain antibiotics, vitamin K dependent factors will decrease. Vitamin K is fat soluble—bile salts produced by liver required for its absorption from intestine. Diseases that interfere with fat absorption, e.g., obstructive jaundice, will produce impaired vitamin K absorption.

The actual clot begins to form in 15 to 20 seconds in severe trauma, and within 1 to 2 minutes in minor vascular trauma. Fibrin forms an interlacing network of threads that traps red blood cells, platelets, and plasma to form a firm clot. The clot occludes the entire lumen of the blood vessel and prevents additional blood loss. Within a few minutes, the clot retracts and pulls the vessel's edges together to further ensure hemostasis. During retraction of the clot, clear straw colored fluid is released from the clot into the circulation. This is serum, which differs from plasma because it does not contain clotting factors and fibrinogen. Serum cannot clot—plasma can.

The coagulation system consists of sequences of proenzymes that circulate in an inactive state in the plasma and are converted to active enzymes when the system is activated. These enzymes, or factors, can be activated in two pathways, the intrinsic and extrinsic coagulation cascade. Two chains, or cascades, have been used to describe the interaction of the coagulation factors that evolve to a final common pathway of clot formation. In effect, each are alternate modes of activating factor X (Table 4–1).

Intrinsic Coagulation System

No direct injury is needed to activate the intrinsic clotting pathway (Fig. 4–3). It is triggered into action by exposure to a foreign substance, usually a collagen surface, resulting from stasis. All factors required for the intrinsic system are present in circulating blood. Intravascular clotting can also be stimulated via the intrinsic pathway by antigen–antibody reactions, direct activation of platelets, circulating debris, platelet aggregation on damaged endothelial linings in vessels, and foreign chemicals, for instance bacterial endotoxins. Conditions such as roughened vessel walls, immune complexes, hemolysis, in addition to blood stasis and bacterial endotoxin can stimulate the intrinsic pathway.

A chain reaction follows until factor X is activated. Once activated, the intrinsic pathway is hard to stop because it perpetuates itself.

Extrinsic Coagulation System

The extrinsic coagulation cascade is stimulated into action by tissue thromboplastin, arising from tissue trauma outside blood vessels (Fig. 4–4). Damaged tissues produce and release thromboplastin, which initiates the clotting cascade to form activated factor X.

Final Common Pathway of Coagulation

Whether the inciting stimulus occurs when the blood comes in contact with an abnormal surface (intrinsic system) or when tissue thromboplastin gains access to the bloodstream (extrinsic system), the final result is the same—the

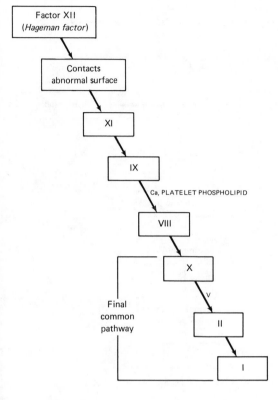

Figure 4-3. Intrinsic coagulation system.

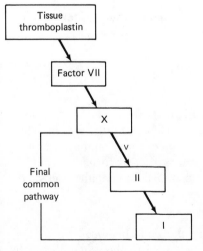

Figure 4-4. Extrinsic coagulation system.

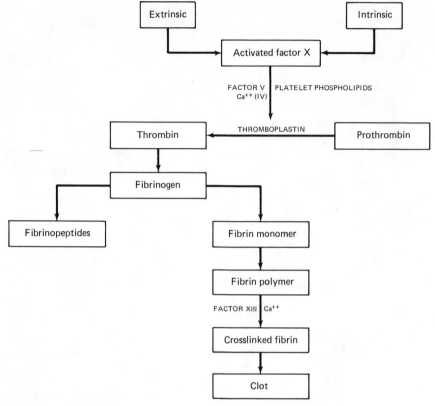

Figure 4-5. Final common pathway of coagulation: Stage III.

production of large amounts of thrombin followed by the transformation of fibrinogen to fibrin. This is called the final common pathway (Fig. 4–5).

ANTICOAGULANT FORCES

A system of checks and balances against widespread clotting is the fibrinolytic system. There are many forces that work on the blood fluidity system. These are regulatory mechanisms or anticoagulant forces that maintain the blood in a fluid state. In the absence of this system, sufficient thrombin could be generated by clotting of only 1 milliliter of blood to coagulate all of the fibrinogen in 3 liters of blood in 15 seconds.

Anticoagulant forces include:

1. The smoothness of the normal vascular endothelium.
2. A layer of negatively charged proteins in the vascular system that repels positively charged clotting factors. Cellular components of circulating

blood are mutually repelled by their electrical charges, remaining separate from one another and from the endothelial lining.

3. Blood flow velocity that promotes dispersion of activated clotting factors and decreases the change of focal fibrin formation. The flow rate is critical and is shown by the absence of fibrin thrombus in patent arteries whereas fibrin thrombus may be massive in venous stasis.

4. Fibrin threads of existing clots absorb 85 to 90 percent of all activated thrombin, containing it within the clot and preventing thrombin from circulating freely in the bloodstream to cause clotting.

5. Antithrombin III, a plasma protein, is believed to inactivate the thrombin that fails to be continued within the clot and neutralizes active clotting enzymes.

6. Heparin, or antithrombin II, is produced by mast cells, which are located primarily in the lungs and liver, and basophils, which are circulating mast cells. Heparin inhibits thrombin and other proteases in the cascade and interferes with the action of thrombin and fibrinogen.

7. Functional capacity of liver and the reticuloendothelial system to produce and filter activated clotting factors that fail to be contained within the clot.

Fibrinolysis is the dissolution of the fibrin clot. It is the physiological process of removing unwanted insoluble fibrin deposits by gradual and progressive enzymatic clearance of fibrin into soluble fragments (Fig. 4–6).

The central event of the fibrinolytic system is the conversion of plasminogen to plasmin. Plasmin digests stabilized fibrin polymers. It can digest fibrinogen, fibrin, prothrombin, and factors V, VIII, and XII.

Four types of substances can convert plasminogen to plasmin:

1. Activation of factor XII—the event that triggers clot formation via activation of factor XII also sets in motion a mechanism for its ultimate resolution.

2. Poorly characterized activators—in lysosomes of the heart, kidney, and other organs, there are activators. At times of extensive organ damage, these activators can be released into the blood. This phenomen may be responsible for frequent occurrence of systemic fibrinolysis in clients with widespread trauma.

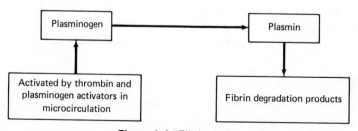

Figure 4-6. Fibrinolysis.

3. Endothelial activators—these are activators present in venous and capillary endothelial cells. They are released into the circulation by physiologic stimuli, for instance exercise; pharmacologic stimuli, for instance nicotinic acid; and pathologic stimuli, for instance hypotensive shock. They are responsible for keeping the microcirculation open and free of fibrin deposits.

4. Fibrinolyte enzymes—urokinase is a substance found in urine that can rapidly transform plasminogen to plasmin. It is not normally found in the circulation but in pathological states, for instance prostatic cancer or extensive urological surgery, it may enter the circulation in pathological amounts and induce systemic fibrinolysis. Streptokinase is a naturally occurring bacterial protein. Both enzymes have been employed in dissolving established thrombi in coronary and pulmonary vessels and in vascular access catheters and devices.

Plasmin digests fibrinogen and breaks down the fibrin thrombi. The clot and other clotting factors are literally dissolved. The dissolution of fibrin thrombi results in fibrin split products (FSP). These products also result from the conversion of fibrinogen to fibrin as part of the clotting process, and they are potent anticoagulants. Once on the scene, FSPs interfere with the clot formation functions of platelets, thrombin, and fibrinogen. Massive intravascular clotting is thus controlled.

The fibrinolytic system may have a role in neoplastic disease. Activity of this system is enhanced when many cell lines undergo virus-induced transformation in culture. The mechanism by which these cells initiate fibrinolysis appears to depend on plasminogen, an activator that is released from the membranes of cells following transformation. Enhanced fibrinolytic activity may be responsible for the morphological appearance of transformed cells and may facilitate metastasis.

THROMBOSIS

Thrombosis is a localized process of vascular occlusion by hemostatic material derived from circulating blood components. It is the response of the hemostatic mechanism to altered endovascular surfaces under variable flow conditions. Thrombus material that breaks away and produces occlusion downstream is a thromboembolus. Thromboses can be generated by vascular injury, difficulties in blood flow, and altered hemostatic mechanisms.

Vascular Injury in Thrombosis

Because normal endothelium presents a nonreactive surface to circulating blood, intimal injury is the main event triggering the thrombotic process. When an artery is injured focally, with exposure of subendothelial structures, platelets immediately accumulate at the site of the injury. Within minutes, a thrombus forms consisting of densely packed platelets, some white cells, and a surrounding fibrin net. Fibrin replaces the platelet mass in about 24 hours. Meanwhile, the thrombus is invaded by neutrophils that phagocytose cellular debris and intact platelets. Therefore, after 2 or 3 days, the amount of fibrin is markedly decreased. By 4 to 7 days, the thrombus is covered with endothelium and contains numerous smooth muscle cells. At the end of a week, the amount of fibrin is further decreased and there is evidence of collagen and elastin formation. A week or so later, the initial platelet mass has organized into a fibrous thickening of the arterial intima, rich in collagen, smooth muscle cells, and elastic fibers.

With injury to smaller vessels, the platelet mass formed at the site of injury readily builds up and breaks down. A platelet mass may be so unstable that it fragments before much fibrin can accumulate or fibrin may be degraded through fibrinolytic activity generated by the intima, leading to fragmentation of the thrombus.

The fresh or evolving arterial thrombus is distinctive because of its predominant platelet composition, the white thrombus. Research suggests that platelet inhibitors may be effective in preventing arterial clots. Arterial thrombi tend to occur at sites of greatest endothelial disruption, for instance around heart valves, downstream from stenoses, at the origin of luminal expansions, lateral to and at the lips of orifices of perpendicular branches, at bifurcations, and on prosthetic surfaces. Microembolization from such thrombotic sites is usual; only the larger, less friable fragments appear to produce emboli that become recognized clinically.

In clients with ongoing arterial thromboembolism, the major role of the platelets in the thrombotic process is selective platelet consumption. Circulating fibrinogen is only minimally consumed in this setting, presumably because procoagulant material is swept away from thrombogenic foci by the rapid arterial flow before coagulation becomes fully activated. Selective platelet consumption is also seen when platelet thromboemboli form on prosthetic surfaces, where the rate of platelet thrombus formation is related to the amount of unendothelialized surface. Interruption of arterial thromboembolism requires inhibition of the platelet function.

Mechanisms causing endothelial injury include physical forces, for instance direct vascular trauma; chemical injury, for instance nicotine, possibly estrogen contraceptives; infectious injury, for instance hemolytic–uremic syndrome; and immune injury.

Blood Flow in Thrombosis

Irregularities in arterial walls produce a turbulent flow pattern that promotes thrombus formation. Platelets collide in such areas of disturbed flow with a likelihood that a platelet mass, once formed, will adhere to the wall. Thrombus formation and atherosclerosis were first associated this way. Atherosclerotic

TABLE 4-2. VARIABLES PROMOTING THROMBOTIC DISEASE

Arterial Factors	Venous Factors
Hypertension	Immobilization
Cigarettes	Trauma
Hyperipidemia	Surgery
Lack of exercise	Malignancy
Obesity	Childbirth
Diabetes	CHF
	↓ Antithrombin

lesions occur principally because of the organization of intravascular fibrin deposits and vascular thrombi. A central hypothesis describing the initiation of atherogenesis and and thrombosis focuses on compromise or injury of the endothelium. Because the endothelium is a nonthrombogenic surface, thrombus formation occurs as a result of endothelial injury. Endothelial damage exposes the underlying subendothelium, a thrombogenic surface. Platelets adhere to the subendothelium and aggregate at the surface. With sufficient endothelial injury, smooth muscle migration and proliferation ensue, which eventually leads to intimal thickening. All of these factors illustrate how a turbulent flow pattern can develop, and predispose the client to thrombus formation. Venous thrombosis typically represents thrombus formation in the presence of static flow and is referred to as red thrombi because it resembles clotted blood.

Altered Hemostatic Mechanisms in Thrombosis

There is an association between arterial thromboembolic disease and increased platelet reactivity (Table 4-2). Venous thromboembolism is increased in clients with increased fibrinogen levels and factors V, VIII, and IX. Also thromboembolic risk is imposed by activation of the coagulation system associated with trauma, surgery, malignancy, and stasis. For instance, brain and lung tissue contains high levels of tissue thromboplastin. If a client has surgery that involves either of these two organs, thromboplastin is released into the the circulation and predisposes to thrombotic disease.

CHAPTER 5
Nursing Care of the Bleeding Client

Hemorrhagic disorders are characterized by abnormal bleeding from defects in hemostatis. Bleeding may be spontaneous or traumatic, localized to one anatomical site or generalized, lifelong or acquired. Although some signs are suggestive of specific hemostatic disorders, nonspecific findings, such as excessive bruising or postoperative hemorrhage, could result from a derangement of virtually any aspect of the hemostatic mechanism.

The formation of a clot results from a finely tuned, orderly progression of events initiated by vascular injury. A myriad of simultaneous events proceeds in a parallel fashion. Those promoting hemostatic plug formation are balanced by events that limit the response. Thus, blood flow dilutes activated clotting factors and plasma inhibitors neutralize them. A fibrinolytic activator released by endothelial cells initiates the process that eventually produces a patent, intact vessel.

Bleeding can result from either a deficiency or a defect of the components needed for hemostatic plug formation or an imbalance between the opposing forces of clot formation and its inhibitor or dissolution. The clot forming potential can be impaired when a sufficient quantity of an individual clotting factor is not available. Many congenital clotting abnormalities are the result of the synthesis of an abnormal protein. In this instance, the plasma contains a normal concentration of a clotting factor that is functionally impaired. There are a number of variations concerning the theme of absent versus deficient coagulation protein synthesis. Some clotting factors have more than one distinct function or enzymatic reaction that can result in several abnormalities. The great majority of acquired coagulation disorders, whether associated with a disease state or resulting from antithrombotic therapy, are complex and involve mutliple clotting factors, clotting factors with platelet disorders, or combinations of factor deficiencies with either fibrinolysis or consumption of coagulation factors. Bleeding and decreased synthesis of coagulation proteins is associated with aberrations of hepatic production of vitamin K dependent factors II, VII, IX, and X and from thrombocytopenia. Bleeding may be caused also by excessive fibrinolysis from antithrombotic therapy or spontaneously.

The complexities of platelet function offer many potential sites for manipulation by pharmacological agents and an equal number of vulnerable loci for malfunction and subsequent hemorrhagic disease. These disorders may result from aberrations in platelet number, function, or accelerated destruction by immune mechanisms and other consumptive process. Thrombocytopenia can result also from decreased production of platelets in the bone marrow. Disturbances in platelet function, which are associated with bleeding, may come about through specific defects in secretion, adhesion, or aggregation. Complex disorders of platelet functions may be acquired as a consequence of a variety of metabolic derangements in which circulating inhibitors of platelet function are present as by-products of the underlying disease.

In the following chapters, many hemostatic disorders are examined in detail. As a common basis for care of patients suffering from these disorders, nursing care of the bleeding client is described here.

CASE STUDY

A 26-year-old man sustained multiple injuries in a motor vehicle accident. His course was complicated with septic shock, adult respiratory distress syndrome, and ultimately disseminated intravascular coagulation (DIC).

Nursing Diagnosis: excessive bleeding/potential for hemorrhage related to DIC as demonstrated by bleeding from IV sites, ecchymoses, and petechiae
Medical Diagnosis: DIC

Outcome. Client's bleeding tendency will be closely monitored.

Nursing Interventions	Rationale	Evaluation
1. Assessment every 1–2 hr for evidence of bleeding. a. note presence of hematuria, bleeding from body orifices or mucous membranes, bleeding from IV sites, other catheters, and nasogastric tubes	Client can potentially lose a significant portion of blood volume through a slow constant ooze as he would with a major hemorrhage. In addition, therapy for a coagulopathy must be constantly evaluated for effectiveness and altered, as necessary.	Client will not demonstrate signs of hypovolemia or anemia from excessive blood loss.

Nursing Interventions	Rationale	Evaluation
b. guaiac (heme-test) all stools, naso-gastric drainage, vomitus, etc.		
c. assess for presence or changes in location and size, of petechiae, purpura, and ecchymoses		
d. measure blood loss as accurately as possible.		
e. check hematocrit—hemoglobin as ordered, and maintain a current type and cross-match		
f. measure abdominal girth every shift		

Outcome. Client will not demonstrate signs of organ failure as a result of thrombi or hemorrhage into organ.

Nursing Interventions	Rationale	Evaluation
Renal		
1. Measure intake and output.	Acute tubular necrosis may develop secondary to thrombi, hemorrhage, or hypovolemia.	Client will have urine output of 30–60 cc-p hr
2. Note changes in client's BUN/creatinine.		
Pulmonary		
3. Assess client every 2 hr for	Respiratory failure may	Client will have a respiratory

Nursing Interventions	Rationale	Evaluation
onset/change in rales, dyspnea, cyanosis, hemoptysis, tachypnea, wheezes. Assist client to cough and deep breathe every 2 hr.	occur due to thrombi, hemor-rhage, or mental status changes.	rate of 20–30 breaths-p min and will have clear breath sounds.

CNS

4. Assess client every 3–4 hr for mental status changes—con-fusion, lethargy, obtundation, coma, seizures.	Cerebral hemor-rhage can result from a bleeding disorder and changes in mental states can occur from thrombi or metabolic dis-turbances.	Client will be alert and ori-ented to time, place, and person.

CV

5. Assess client for changes in BP and peripheral perfusion—color and temperature of extremities, presence of pulses, presence of acral cynosis.	Shock can be caused by fibrin being rampantly deposited in the microcirculation and return of blood to the right heart is decreased, lead-ing to a de-creased cardiac output. The presence of shock with a high central venous pressure and signs of pul-monary edema may occur as a result of clotting in the lungs. Coagulopathies and immobility predispose the	Client will have stable vital signs. Extremities will be warm, pink with pulses present.
6. Access every 4 hr for neck vein distention, abnormal heart sounds.		
7. Check Homan's sign every 4 hr and report any calf tenderness on dorsiflexion of the foot.		
8. Assist with range of motion.		

Nursing Interventions	Rationale	Evaluation
	client to thromboembolic disease.	
Psychosocial		
9. Explain all polices, treatment with procedures at client's level of of understanding. Incorporate family members. Allow time for questions with answers.	Stress has been implicated in activation of the fibrinolytic system.	Client will report no feelings of panic or fear.
10. Incorporate use of relaxation techniques, biofeedback, and imagery to decrease stress levels.		

Outcome. Client will not be exposed to situations that cause him to bleed.

Nursing Interventions	Rationale	Evaluation
1. Institute bleeding precautions.	Trauma, even in a mild form, can precipitate bleeding.	Client will not bleed from orifices or catheter sites.
a. avoid rectal temperatures		
b. avoid shaving with a straight blade, use only electric razors		
c. avoid intramuscular or subcutaneous injections.		
d. check blood pressure by cuff as infrequently as possible		
e. use only paper or		

Nursing Interventions	Rationale	Evaluation
silk tape to stabilize catheters and lines		
f. avoid trauma to the mucuous membranes by:		
i. using foam swabs to clean teeth and gums in place of a toothbrush		
ii. avoid foods highly spiced or high in roughage		
iii. avoid use of ill-fitting dentures		
iv. if an indwelling catheter or tube is in place, secure it to client with tape to avoid putting tension on mucous membrane		
v. lubricate all tubes and catheters well		
vi. avoid vaginal and rectal suppositories (Table 5–1)		
2. Use gentleness in all nursing care.		
3. Mouth care every 3–4 hr, using mild solution of saline, bicarbonate, or peroxide.	Because ischemia is common in the mouth, client needs frequent mouth care. Conventional mouth-wash too drying to mucous membranes.	Client's oral mucous membranes and teeth will be free of clots and debris.

Nursing Interventions	Rationale	Evaluation
4. Keep skin well lubricated by: a. maintaining high humidity in client's room b. frequent application of lubricant 5. Avoid use of aspirin and aspirin containing drugs.	Skin should be well lubricated to prevent drying of skin and subsequent cracking.	Client's skin will be moist and intact.

TABLE 5-1. BLEEDING PRECAUTIONS

Avoid use of	Do
1. Rectal temps 2. Razors 3. IM or SC injections 4. A diet high in roughage or spicy food 5. Ill-fitting dentures 6. Mouthwash 7. Rectal/vaginal suppositories 8. Aspirin	1. Check BP by cuff as infrequently as possible. 2. Use only paper/silk tape to stabilize catheters. 3. Use foam swab, in place of tooth-brush, for dental care. 4. Lubricate tubes and catheters well. 5. Maintain a current type and cross-match. 6. Observe for signs and symptoms of bleeding. 7. Test all urine, stool, and emesis for blood.

CHAPTER 6
Alterations in Protective Mechanisms: Bleeding Disorders

DISSEMINATED INTRAVASCULAR COAGULATION

Disseminated intravascular coagulation (DIC) is not a new syndrome. It was first observed more than a 100 years ago when an investigator discovered gross intravascular coagulation of animal blood following an infusion of hemolyzed erythrocytes. DIC is a pathological syndrome that is always secondary to other diseases. Patients with DIC are often critically ill because of their primary problem. It is a unique disorder of coagulation during which hemorrhage and thrombosis occur simultaneously. This chapter describes the current understanding of the pathological mechanisms and their relationship to the diseases that underlie this syndrome.

The overall process in DIC is a consequence of the formation of thrombin. Thrombin catalyzes the activation and the subsequent consumption of certain coagulant proteins and the production of fibrin. Fibrin is deposited in the microcirculation, depleting the body of essential clotting components. This results in consumption coagulopathy. Clots form where they are not needed, and indeed where they are harmful—in the microcirculation, especially the skin and the kidneys—yet, clots cannot form at the injury site. The presence of thrombin in plasma activates the fibrinolytic system, resulting in excessive fibrinolysis and more bleeding. Clinically, these manifestations are also influenced by the diseased state that triggers DIC (Table 6–1).

Etiology. DIC is inappropriate, accelerated, and systemic activation of the coagulation cascade. Alteration of any of the components of the vascular system, namely vessel wall, plasma proteins, and platelets can result in DIC (Fig. 6–1).

There appear to be two major mechanisms under which the multiple inciting etiologies of DIC can be categorized: endothelial injury and tissue injury. Endothelial injury relates to those disease states that specifically injure the endothelium with resultant kallikrein–kinin system activation e.g., infec-

TABLE 6-1. DISEASES ASSOCIATED WITH DIC

Neoplasm	Leukemias
	Solid tumors especially lung, prostate, and breast
OB	Amniotic fluid embolus
	Abruptio placenta
Immunological	Incompatible blood transfusion, graft versus host disease
	Anaphylaxis, thrombocytopenia, immune complex disease
Congenital	Hyaline membrane disease, sickle cell anemia
Infection	Septic shock, malaria
Metabolic/Endocrine	Diabetic ketoacidosis, acute fatty liver, adrenal and renal disease
Circulatory	Prolonged cardiopulmonary bypass, malignant hyperthermia, shock, and pulmonary emboli
Trauma	Burns
	Extensive Surgery
	Fat emboli
	ECMO
	Snake bite
Respiratory	ARDS
	Anoxia

tions. Tissue injury refers to those disease states (e.g., malignancy) in which procoagulant material is released into the circulation. In addition, there are modulating cellular and extracellular systems that extend or limit the reactions, thereby modifying the manifestations of DIC.

Injury or extensive alteration to the vascular endothelium exposes the basement membrane. Collagen alone or in combination with other connective tissue components and platelet factors then activates factor XII. This activates the intrinsic coagulation system, the fibrinolytic system, and the kinin formation. Kinin formation results from the activation of factor XII of prekallikrein to kallikrein, which then liberates bradykinin. Bradykinin produces vasodilation. DIC due to the intrinsic coagulation system activation is almost always accompanied by hypotension, which can be attribute to the bradykinin release. Hypotension is a unique feature of DIC associated with the intrinsic system activation and distinguishes it from DIC associated with tissue injury. Some pathological conditions, which lead to activation of the intrinsic coagulation system, include prolonged cardiopulmonary bypass, amniotic fluid emboli, anoxia, shock, and adult respiratory distress syndrome (ARDS).

The intrinsic sytem can be activated also by damage to the RBCs, with subsequent release of procoagulants that activate factor XII. Examples of this phenomenon include malaria, sickle cell anemia, transfusion reactions, and endotoxemia. Gram-negative endotoxins may be the most common of DIC. They act directly on factor XII and initiate the intrinsic system. Endotoxin

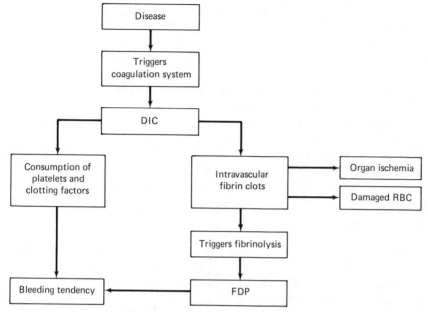

Figure 6-1. Pathophysiology of DIC.

can also initiate DIC by producing clumping of blood cells in the microcirculation.

Tissue injury, with the resultant release of coagulant material into the circulation, is the second major initiating mechanism of DIC. Tissue injury activates the extrinsic system of coagulation releasing tissue thromboplastin into the blood. Studies show that tissue thromboplastin injected into animals consistently causes incoagulable blood. Tissue thromboplastin leads to the ultimate conversion of prothrombin to thrombin.

The triggering mechanism of DIC in neoplastic disorders appears to be the release of coagulant proteins from the tumor. This hypothesis is supported by the fact that chemotherapy can aggravate the DIC in leukemia. Tissue thromboplastic activity is higher in malignant tissues than in the normal tissues, but more specific coagulants may also be involved. The most common neoplasms which lead to the release of tissue thromboplastin and predispose the client to DIC are leukemia, pancreatic and prostatic adenocarcinoma, and lung and brain tumors, but a wide variety of tumors appear to predispose to the development of DIC.

DIC can be triggered by the release of tissue thromboplastin as a result of surgery. For example, during transurethral prostatectomy, irrigation transports tissue fluids into the circulation; moreover, if distilled water is used, it causes the hemolysis of viable cells. Prostatic tissue is rich in proteolytic enzymes and plasminogen activators, and therefore, operations involving this type of tissue are commonly associated with laboratory evidence of DIC and occasionally, clinical manifestations.

Platelet and red blood cell injury has been considered to accelerate DIC, due to the release of phospholipids. Clients with DIC have been noted to have a decreased reticuloendothelial system (RES) clearing function, thereby aggravating the process by limiting the removal of activated clotting factors. Recent evidence suggests that decreased tissue macrophage function may be due to a decreased circulating opsonin, fibronectin. Fibronectin mediates reticuloendothelial or macrophage clearance of particulate matter such as fibrin clumps, collagen debris, and bacterial products. Fibronectin is reported to be decreased, presumably due to cross-linking with fibrin in patients with DIC and low levels correlated with poor prognosis. It is unknown whether decreased fibronectin is secondary to, or responsible for, the clinical outcome in these patients.

Pathophysiology. Both the intrinsic and extrinsic systems are triggering mechanisms that liberate free thrombin into the circulation and produce clotting. Thrombin, in addition to converting fibrinogen to fibrin and ultimately fibrin clots, causes platelet aggregation. These clumps of platelets are part of the thrombotic component of DIC and may lead to organ impairment. During thrombin generation, prothrombin and other procoagulants, especially factors II, V, and VII, are depleted. This produces a hemorrhagic tendency by depleting the body of fibrinogen, platelets, and clotting factors.

The formation of the fibrin clot then activates the fibrinolytic system. Plasmin, or fibrinolysin, is produced to dissolve or lyse the clot. Plasmin is a proteolytic enzyme that digests fibrin, fibrinogen, factors V, VII, XII, and prothrombin. Products known as fibrin split products (FSPs) or fibrin degradation products (FDPs) are released from the widespread fibrinolysis. FSPs are potent anticoagulants. Normally, they are removed from the circulation by the RES. In DIC, fibrinolytic agents and FSPs continue to circulate in the body, and cause more bleeding.

There is normally a delicate balance between coagulation, fibrinolysis, and the function of the RES in maintaining hemostasis. DIC occurs when coagulation mechanisms are abnormally stimulated.

Clinical Presentation. DIC is the symptom of a disease process that may have many different causes. Because the diagnosis of DIC depends initially on clinical suspicion, it is critical to discover all of the factors that initiate, predispose, or maintain DIC in each client.

Widespread clot formation occurs in capillaries in the microcirculation and causes decreased nutritional flow to body cells. This inappropriate clotting results from the presence of thrombin in the systemic circulation, which results in fibrin deposition in small vessels. The decreased nutritional flow to the tissues leads to tissue ischemia, or lack of oxygen and nutrients. It is most pronounced in the kidneys, lungs, brain, gastrointestinal (GI) tract, pancreas, adrenals, and pituitary gland. Diffuse clotting leads to the depletion of clotting factors. Platelet aggregation decreases the number of active circulating platelets and results in thrombocytopenia.

The secondary activation of the fibrinolytic system follows the liberation of plasminogen activator from disrupted cell lysosomes and widespread fibrin formation. Fibrin is degraded by plasmin, leading to FSP formation. FSPs are strong anticoagulants that inhibit thrombin formation and decrease platelet aggregation, potentiating the hemorrhagic tendencies. In some cases, fibrin may remain in the microcirculation long enough to damage red blood cells flowing through the fibrin mesh. Formation of schistocytes or fragmented red blood cells results.

Nursing Assessments. Clinically, the client will bleed, whether in an occult or an overt form. Knowing that the common factors that predispose to DIC are hypotension, stasis of capillary blood, hypoxemia, and acidosis, the nurse should observe for signs and symptoms of bleeding in any client with these clinical problems. Manifestations may include purpura, hemorrhagic bullae, wound hematomas, gangrene, widespread ecchymosis, and petechiae. Note oozing of blood from mucous membranes, needle puncture sites, and incisions. Occult hemorrhage may be in the form of abdominal distention, guaiac positive stool or emesis, hematuria, changes in skin of sclera color, malaise, weakness, altered sensorium, vision changes, headaches, air hunger, orthopnea, tachycardia, or acrocyanosis. Acrocyanosis, a sharp irregular demarcation of cyanosis on the periphery, results from fibrin deposited in the microcirculation. It is diagnostic for DIC and can lead to tissue necrosis and gangrene.

If DIC occurs slowly and chronically, as it happens with some carcinomas, the clinical picture is that of emboli problems or troublesome minor episodes of bleeding.

Impaired tissue perfusion can demonstrate itself in many ways: restlessness, confusion, abnormal behavior, decreased urine output, ST changes, syncope, hemiplegia, dyspnea, tachypnea, pulmonary emboli, and organ necrosis, especially acute tubular necrosis. Sudden massive hemorrhage is not infrequent. Gastrointestinal and genitourinary bleeding and respiratory tract hemorrhage are possible. The client may exhibit signs of thrombotic vasular occlusion (Fig. 6–2).

Laboratory Studies. Diagnosis can be difficult. Multiple transfusions may dilute plasma coagulation factors or platelets. Liver disease with portal hypertension can cause decreased plasma coagulation factors, thrombocytopenia, and activation of the fibrinolytic system. Thrombocytopenia may arise from many other causes.

The laboratory diagnosis of DIC is made by a decreased platelet count and fibrinogen level and a prolonged prothrombin time in the presence of a hemorrhagic or thrombotic state (Table 6–2).

Thrombocytopenia is a cardinal feature of DIC and in about half of the

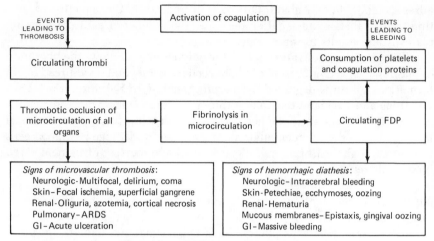

Figure 6-2. Sequence of events—DIC.

cases the platelet counts are below 50,000. Low plasma fibrinogen is due to a combination of consumption by thrombin-induced clotting and plasmin-induced fibrinolysis. The prolonged prothrombin time reflects the decrease in factor V and, to a lesser extent, factors II, X, and fibrinogin. However, the diagnosis of DIC requires the measurment of FSPs or FDPs.

Medical Interventions. The most effective treatment is to correct the primary disorder. General supportive measures, such as fluid replacement and maintenance of adequate oxygenation and blood pressure, are indicated. A clinical judgment of the client's immediate response to these therapeutic measures, that is, whether they will sustain the client, curtail the complicating DIC process, and allow for reasonably rapid, spontaneous recovery, is the major factor in deciding upon additional treatment. Thus, life threatening or progressive, severe microvascular occlusions due to DIC would warrant interruption of thrombosis by heparin anticoagulation, and serious hemorrhagic manifestations would require subsequent aggressive replacement treatment with platelets and plasma clotting factors.

Heparin is administered primarily to inhibit the formation of microthrombi, even though the dominant clinical feature may be hemorrhage. The dose of heparin should be therapeutic, that is, adequate to overcome the prothrombotic forces.

Heparin interferes with the coagulation cascade at several sites. It antagonizes the production of thrombin and aborts the clotting process by preventing clot formation and secondary activation of the fibrinolytic system. It inhibits clot formation but has no effect on formed clots. In DIC, it is used to interrupt intravascular generation of thrombin and further deposition of fibrin

TABLE 6-2. LABORATORY DATA IN DIC

Test	Normal Range	DIC	Comment
Prothrombin time (PT)	12–15 sec	> 15 sec *or* > 5 sec over patient's usual value *or* 4 sec + control	Test of extrinsic system Prolonged in DIC, liver disease, vitamin K deficiency, or coumarin therapy
Fibrinogen	150–350 mg/dl	< 150 mg/dl *or* when level ↓ 150 mg/dl from patients usual level	↓ DIC, liver disease. Patients with chronic disease have ↑ fibrinogen. For these patients, a fall in fibrinogen to 200 mg/dl can be misleading if taken in isolation
Platelets	250,000–500,000	< 150,000 *or* a ↓ of 200,000	Chemotherapy
Fibrin split products (FSP)	< 10 mg/ml	> 40 mg/ml	↓ DIC, liver disease ↑ DIC, liver disease
Thrombin time	15 sec	20–40 sec	↑ DIC, liver disease
Partial prothrombin time	39–53 sec	> 10 sec + control	Test of intrinsic system Prolonged in DIC, Hemophilia, and heparin therapy
Clotting factors	> 80%	10–40%	With most factors, clotting occurs normally if factor levels > 15% ↓ V + VIII—DIC ↓ V + X—Liver disease (normal VIIII) ↓ X + ↑ PT, PTT—Vitamin K deficiency
Peripheral blood smear		Shistocytes	Distorted RBC by passing through fibrin matrix

in the microcirculation. It also prevents agglutination of platelets. The goal of heparin therapy is to tip the balance within the microcirculation toward physiologic fibrinolysis and allow reperfusion of the skin, kidneys, and brain. Although heparin may stop the clotting process, it may worsen the bleeding. The use of heparin should be avoided, or used with caution, when bleeding continues because of the anticoagulant effects of FDPs and not because of the consumption of factors, or because of a defect in the vasculature, or because of a severe fibrin deficiency.

Heparin dosage is generally regulated to double the total blood clotting time, or to get the partial prothrombin time (PTT) to 2½ times normal. A bolus intravenous injection of 10,000 units or more could then be followed by intermittent intravenous injections or continuous intravenous administration. As logic would dictate, the bleeding could be worsened initially by the effect of heparin. Therefore, immediately after the institution of heparin, the bleeding diathesis should be treated by replenishing the depleted (consumed) supply of platelets and clotting factors using platelet concentrate and fresh-frozen plasma or cryoprecipitate.

Clinical effectiveness of the therapy is determined by monitoring plasma fibrinogen concentration and platelet counts. Any increase in platelet counts or plasma fibrinogen concentration is an encouraging indication that the consumption process has been interrupted and bleeding is under control. Transfusion without prior administration of heparin adds fuel to the fire of thrombosis and does not effectively correct the plasma deficiency state. Clients with DIC frequently require inordinately large amounts of heparin to overcome intravascular coagulation.

Heparin can lead to major thrombus formation with the formation of antiplatelet antibodies. This can happen after 8 days on heparin therapy. The nurse should keep a careful check on the platelet count. Continuous infusions of heparin are less likely to cause significant bleeding. Side effects may include hemorrhage and anaphylaxis.

The role of fibrinolytic inhibitors in DIC is limited and they should be used with caution in such patients. An excessive concentration of FDPs in the blood may contribute to the hemorrhagic diathesis, and the rationale for using inhibitors is to decrease their concentration by curtailing the lysis of microthrombin. The indication for use should not be a laboratory value, no matter how abnormal, but rather a clinical state of dangerous, excessive, or extremely bothersome bleeding that has not responded to replacement treatment and that hampers care and threatens life.

One drug that can be used is aminocaproic acid (Epsilon-Aminocaproic Acid). This antifibrinolytic drug retards the lysis of clots where clots are appropriate and slows bleeding. It does, however, carry the risk of impending lysis of inappropriate clots in vital tissue. Concomitant administration of heparin may counteract this effect.

Nursing Interventions. The nurse should institute bleeding precautions (see Chap. 5). The client's laboratory values, especially PT/PTT, bleeding times, and platelets should be closely monitored to assess the effects of therapy. Blood products may be required and the nurse should administer those with the appropriate safety measures (see the section on Transfusion Therapy). The client may be in multisystem failure, and the nurse needs to plan care for him in accordance to the client's other needs.

VON WILLEBRAND'S DISEASE

Von Willebrand's disease (VWB) is an autosomal, dominant or recessive hereditary disorder existing in three forms, depending on the particular biochemical defect. It is a deficiency in factor VIII, the clotting protein essential for normal functioning of the intrinsic cascade and for normal adhesion of platelets to hemostatic sites. Therefore, a client with VWB has abnormalities in platelet adhesion and in function of the intrinsic cascade.

VWB is the congenital bleeding disorder most commonly diagnosed in adult life; along with hemophilias A and B, it comprises the majority of inherited hemorrhagic diseases. Its true incidence is difficult to establish because mild cases do not come to the attention of a physician. No racial or ethnic incidence has been reported.

Pathophysiology. VWB may result from an absence or a decrease in factor VIII or from its presence in inactive form. Laboratory studies demonstrate that the clotting disorder may result from impaired platelet adhesion to the vessel wall.

VWB can be inherited in a number of ways. Recessive VWB inherited from both parents is usually clinically and biologically very severe. A carrier of VWB will be asymptomatic with normal bleeding times and factor VIII. VWB type I is transmitted as an autosomal dominant trait and is characterized by variably decreased levels of factor VIII. Bleeding time is usually prolonged. VWB type II is also transmitted as an autosomal dominant trait but is characterized by an absence of factor VIII. Subtypes II A and II B show variable laboratory findings and are inherited as recessive traits. A few cases of acquired VWB have been reported. In such cases there is sudden onset of bleeding symptoms in clients with previously normal hemostasis. There may be an immunological basis for acquired VWB.

Clinical Presentation. Clients with clinically significant bleeding are commonly seen in health care settings. In most clients, bleeding is due to a local cause rather than a generalized hemostatic defect. The diagnostic problem is to determine whether or not the client is bleeding as a result of local factors or a generalized hemostatic defect.

A careful history should be obtained from the client. The client may describe bleeding from multiple sites. Is his bleeding spontaneous, taking the form of petechiae, hematomas, large bruises, or hemarthrosis? Is bleeding after minor trauma disproportionately severe? A client with VWB may describe symptoms from infancy or early childhood and will often have a family history of bleeding in response to previous operations or trauma.

In severe VWB, the onset of bleeding typically occurs in early childhood and tends to decrease with age. In moderate or mild forms, a bleeding tendency may not be apparent before adulthood.

Nursing Assessments. Bleeding may be manifested in a number of ways. Mucosal and cutaneous hemorrhages are the most frequent, including epistaxis, gingival bleeding, bleeding from inflamed tonsils, and bruising; menorrhagia is very frequent and excessive postpartum bleeding occurs in about one third of the cases. Gastrointestinal bleeding is not infrequent and is often without identifiable cause. Excessive bleeding following tonsillectomy, other surgery, or dental extraction is common in the absence of replacement therapy and has often led to the diagnosis of the disease. Muscular hematoma and hemarthrosis are rare.

A careful assessment of previous response to trauma is important. Specific inquiries should be made about bleeding from the umbilical cord after birth and bleeding after circumcision, tooth extractions, tonsillectomy, and abdominal operations. If tonsillectomy or major abdominal operations have been tolerated without excessive blood loss, it is unlikely that the client is suffering from a severe disorder. A family history usually reveals that at least 50 percent of the family members are affected in some way.

Examine the client for spontaneous subcutaneous and mucous membrane hemorrhage, petechiae, and other superficial forms of bleeding. Bleeding usually starts within seconds after injury and continues for hours but once it stops, it does not usually recur.

Physical examination of clients with hemorrhagic disorders should include a detailed assessment of the sites of bleeding.

Laboratory Studies. Laboratory values that are abnormal in VWB are: bleeding time, factor VIII levels, and platelet adhesivity tests. A prolonged bleeding time is one of the most important criteria for diagnosis of VWB. It is always prolonged at some time in the course of the disease. Detection of a factor VIII deficiency is measured immunologically by electroimmunodiffusion. Platelet adhesivity is measured by the use of ristocetin-induced platelet aggregation in platelet-rich plasma. Ristocetin is an antibiotic found to aggregate platelets in a platelet-rich plasma in normal individuals. Platelet adhesivity is decreased. PTT is long, caused by a low level of factor VIII.

Medical Interventions. Transfusion therapy in the form of cryoprecipitate is administered for bleeding episodes and prophylactically 1 day prior to surgery. Cryoprecipitate is a solution of factor VIII, fibrinogen, and fibronectin. In severe bleeding episodes, the dose of cryoprecipitate should be adjusted to correct the bleeding time. After cryoprecipitate administration, the client will have normal levels of factor VIII polymer as deposited on any subendothelial surface exposed to injured blood vessels. This leads to an increased platelet adherence, decreased bleeding time, and decreased bleeding. The effects last approximately 4 hours and will need to be readministered if bleeding continues. Local measures to stop bleeding are indicated also. In some types of VWB, the client may be helped by an analogue of vasopressin (antidiuretic hormone). This agent may induce endothelial cells to release their stores of factor VIII.

Nursing Interventions. Client teaching is aimed at prevention of injury and cessation of bleeding when injury occurs. The client should be aware of the fact that he is prone to hemorrhage due to a missing clotting factor, and needs to take precautions against exposing himself to injury. These precautions include wearing shoes at all times, using a soft toothbrush, using an electric razor, and avoidance of puncture wounds. He should recognize and report early signs of bleeding including bruising. The use of aspirin and aspirin-containing products should be avoided. The nurse should also instruct the client on local measures to stop bleeding once it occurs including the application of pressure for at least 5 minutes and to seek assistance for transfusion therapy if these measures are ineffective. In addition, the client should advise dentists or other health care practitioners of his bleeding disorder so cryoprecipitate will be given prophylactically. His condition may precipitate feelings of helplessness and fear, and this can develop into severe self-imposed restrictions on his activities. Consistent teaching and realistic reassurance can prevent these reactions.

HEMOPHILIA

Hemophilia (H) is a hereditary bleeding disorder resulting from deficiencies of specific clotting factors. Classic hemophilia (HA) results from a deficiency of factor VIII. It accounts for 80 percent of the clients with hemophilia. Christmas disease (HB) is a deficiency of factor IX, and accounts for 15 percent of the cases.

Hemophilia has a 1 in 10,000 incidence. It is an X-linked recessive trait. Female carriers transmit genes for hemophilia to half of their daughters who become carriers, and to half of their sons, who develop overt hemophilia.

Pathophysiology. Classic hemophilia HA is, with rare exception, a disease of men, all of whose sons will be normal and all of whose daughters will be obligatory carriers of the trait. Because of the high mutation rate for this disease, as many as one-third of hemophiliacs have no family members with demonstrable evidence or history of coagulopathy.

The defect in HA is a molecular defect on factor VIII, whereas in HB, it is a molecular deficit on factor IX. The clinical picture with HA or HB is identical. The client will have abnormal bleeding because of an absence, or deficiency in, the specific clotting factor. A hemophiliac forms a platelet plug at the bleeding site but the clotting factor deficiency impairs his hemostatic response and capacity to form a stable fibrin clot. This produces abnormal bleeding, which may be mild, moderate, or severe, depending on the degree of factor deficiency.

Clinical Presentations. The clinical hallmarks of both hemophilias A and B are: lack of excessive hemorrhage from minor cuts or abrasions, due to the normalcy of platelet function; joint and muscle hemorrhages that lead to the most difficult and disabling long-term sequelae; easy bruising; prolonged and potentially fatal postoperative hemorrhage; and a panoply of social, psychological, vocational, and economic problems.

Nursing Assessments. The client will describe a variable history dependent on the severity of the disease. Clients with mild hemophilia demonstrate easy bruising, hematomas, nosebleeds, and prolonged bleeding after minor surgery. It can be overlooked into adulthood. Severe hemophiliacs describe spontaneous bleeding and severe bleeding after minor trauma. They also describe large subcutaneous and deep intramuscular hematoma formation. The client with severe hemophilia may have a number of variable symptoms and signs, secondary to bleeding near peripherial nerves or into joints. A detailed family history is necessary to definitively diagnose hemophilia.

Physical assessment can reveal joint pain, swelling, or permanent deformity due to bleeding. The joints most frequently involved are, in descending order of frequency, knees, elbows, ankles, shoulders, hips, and wrists. The first episodes of bleeding into joints, or hemarthrosis, occur in childhood, but often not until the child begins to walk. Hemarthrosis is usually either spontaneous or associated with imperceptible trauma. The onset of hemorrhage is signaled by an "aura," consisting of a vague warmth, tingling sensation, and a sense of mild restlessness or anxiety. This aura may last up to 2 hours. Mild discomfort and slight limitation of joint motion occur next followed (after one to several hours) by pain, joint swelling, cutaneous warmth, and eventual severe limitation of motion. Once bleeding has stopped, the blood is resorbed and the joint returns to normal over several days to several weeks. When pain, swelling, and severe limitation of motion are present, the hemorrhage is far advanced and the process of synovitis begins; this may predispose the joint to further episodes of hemarthrosis and to hemophilia arthropathy. Joint hemorrhage should be treated at the earliest symptoms, long before the development of any physical findings, to prevent the long-term disabling sequelae. Adults may demonstrate periodic joint pain due to established hemophilic arthropathy rather than bleeding; may have considerable fibrosis of the joint capsule, thus preventing joint swelling; may develop chronic limitation of motion, thus removing the value of this finding; and may exhibit defense mechanisms including repression or denial of the existence of hemorrhage.

Hemophilic arthropathy is a major disabling lesion in these clients. With each episode of major hemarthrosis, inflammatory and hypertrophic changes occur in the synovial tissue, sometimes as soon as 4 days after major hemarthrosis. Inflamed and enzyme-producing synovial tissue, erythrocyte debris, and leukocytes all contribute to the erosion of cartilage and bone. Proliferative chronic synovitis also leads to the presence of highly vascular tissue at or near articulating surfaces, thus increasing the frequency of repeated hemorrhages. This vicious cycle leads to the destruction of cartilage, resorption of bone, and formation of bone cysts that communicate with joint space. Anatomical instability of joints also leads to more frequent hemorrhages within the joint itself as well as in neighboring joints and muscles. Finally, chronic pain with subsequent disuse atrophy of local muscle groups occurs with fibrosis of large joints.

Small intramuscular hemorrhages are common but large hematomas may lead to severe sequelae by way of compression of vital structures. Large hematomas may produce fever, leukocytosis, severe pain, and hyperbilirubinemia due to red blood cell degradation.

Hematuria is common and usually painless. Mild flank pain may be present. Intracranial bleeding accounts for 25 percent of the deaths in hemophiliacs in one-half of whom antecedent trauma has occurred. Bleeding may be subdural, epidural, intracerebral, subarachnoid, or rarely intraspinal. Other sites of hemorrhage include gastrointestinal, gingival, or nosebleeds. Bleeding near peripheral nerves can cause peripheral neuropathies, pain, paresthesias, and muscle atrophy.

Laboratory Studies. Clients with HA have a factor VIII assay of 0 to 30 percent of normal, a prolonged PTT, and normal platelets, bleeding time and PT. Clients with HB have a deficient factor IX assay, a prolonged PT and coagulation results similar to HA.

In HA or HB the degree of factor deficiency determines the clinical severity. Mild hemophilia is caused by factor levels of 25 to 50 percent of normal; moderate by factor levels of 5 to 25 percent of normal, and severe in less than 1 percent of normal.

Medical Interventions. The priority is to stop the bleeding. In HA, the client is given antihemophilia factor (AHF) to bring the clotting levels up to 25 percent or more of normal. AHF is a concentrate of factor VIII. AHF only lasts 10 to 12 hours therefore repeat transfusions are needed until the bleeding stops. The minimum hemostatic level of factor VIII for relatively mild hemorrhages is 30 percent, whereas for advanced joint or muscle bleeding or other major hemorrhagic lesions it is 50 percent. One to several days of maintenance therapy are needed for such advanced lesions to resolve, this is achieved by repeating the infusion at 24-hour intervals at approximately 75 percent of the original dose infused. For life threatening lesions or surgery, 80 to 100 percent should be achieved and the factor VIII level kept above 30 to 50 percent by means of appropriate doses of factor VIII infused at intervals of 8 to 12 hours.

AHF is obtained from pooled, citrated fresh-frozen human plasma. A risk does exist that the client may contract acquired immune deficiency syndrome (AIDS) from the AHF. Clients should be aware of this risk, with appropriate teaching and reassurance provided. The incidence of contracting AIDS from AHF is extremely small.

Wet-frozen cryoprecipitate was the product of choice several years ago for bleeding episodes and is still used in some centers. It should be used preferentially when the client has mild hemophilia and seldom requires exposure to blood products (to minimize the risk of hepatitis). For clients with moderately severe hemophilia, plasma product requirements are such that abnormalities of liver function tests appear to be as frequent with cryoprecipitate as with commercial concentrates.

Cryoprecipitate is obtained from fresh-frozen plasma after slow thawing. Each 10-to 40-cc bag of cryoprecipitate contains about 70 to 100 units of factor VIII. Treatment requiring 1500 units of factor VIII should, therefore, use between 15 and 21 bags of cryoprecipitate. The disadvantages of cryoprecipitate include its inconvenience for home use (because of storage at very low temperatures), long preparation time, and the unreliability of its factor VIII content.

There are now available numerous commercial factor VIII concentrates that are made from large pools of normal plasma, sold in lyophilized form and reconstituted as efficient sources of factor VIII. These products allow accurate dose calculations, are convenient for home use, are stable at home refrigeration temperatures for weeks to months, and can be rapidly prepared for self-administration. The major disadvantage is cost.

Local measures to control bleeding are necessary. Ice bags should be applied to the injured part, and thrombin soaked fibrin sponges can be applied to the wound. Activity should be restricted for 48 hours to prevent rebleeding. Elevate the joint, if it has been bled into. It may be immobilized and the blood aspirated. Pain control is necessary.

For bleeding episodes in clients with HB, replacement of factor IX is necessary. The survival time of factor IX is considerably longer than for factor VIII, approximately 24 hours. The minimum hemostatic level is 10 to 25 percent. For major bleeding, a factor IX level of 40 percent should be achieved. Plasma is still used as a source of factor IX when bleeding is minor or in clients not extensively exposed to plasma products. Prothrombin complex concentrates are the major treatment source for clients with severe HB.

Clients may develop side effects from replacement therapy. Occasionally, they develop allergic reactions to cryoprecipitate, manifested as urticaria, pruritis, low grade fever, or bronchospasm. The major side effect of cryoprecipitate or factor VIII concentrate is hepatitis. The majority of treated hemophiliacs will have plasma levels of hepatitis B surface antibody and significant minority (2 to 4 percent) will carry hepatitis B surface antigen. The incidence of overt clinical hepatitis is low.

Administration of large doses of factor IX concentrate has been associated with the development of deep venous thrombosis and pulmonary embolus, especially in settings known to predispose to venous thrombosis, such as the postoperative state or in clients with liver disease. Another major side effect is hepatitis.

Nursing Interventions. Clients with hemophilia require comprehensive nursing care to maximize their health status. Teaching about the nature of the disease and the transmission pattern is important. Consultation with a geneticist for genetic screening is recommended if the client's parents intend to have more children. The client should be aware of: how to recognize a bleeding episode; which measures he should institute first; and how to differentiate between an episode that can be controlled at home versus one that requires hospital care. The side effects of replacement therapy should be well understood by the client and reassurance given about the small possibility of contracting AIDS.

PLATELET DISORDERS

Thrombocytopenia or platelet counts of less than 200,000 can be caused by many factors. One cause is decreased production of platelets. Decreased platelet production can be secondary to: administration of certain drugs such as cytotoxic agents, gold, sulfonamides, and ethanol; irradiation of the bone marrow; generalized decrease in production of all marrow cells, for instance in aplastic anemia; marrow replacement or infiltration as in marrow fibrosis, leukemia, and metastatic carcinoma; and maturation disorders where the bone marrow shows a normal or increased number of megakaryocytes but thrombopoiesis is ineffective from vitamin B_{12} or folate deficiency or myeloproliferative disorders.

Thrombocytopenia can also be due to an increased destruction of platelets secondary to: autoantibody mediated platelet injury such as in autoimmune thrombocytopenic purpura and systemic lupus erythematous; alloantibodies associated with pregnancy or transfusions; DIC due to in vivo thrombin activity and increased rate of destruction; antibodies associated with the use of drugs such as quinidine, quinine, and sulfonamides; and hypersplenism that causes sequestration of platelets. With massive splenomegaly, up to 80 percent of the platelets may be stored in the spleen. Thrombocytopenia can be due to other causes, for instance infections, malfunctioning prosthetic cardiac valves, and thrombotic thrombocytopenia purpura.

With a platelet count of over 40,000, the client will have no spontaneous bleeding, but may bleed after surgery. Between 10,000 and 40,000 platelets, spontaneous bleeding of a mild degree is common. With a platelet count of less than 10,000, bleeding is severe. Spontaneous bleeding is in the form of petechiae, purpuric spots, and confluent ecchymoses. It may occur from any mucous membrane including nose and uterus, GI tract, urinary tract, and respiratory tract.

SPECIFIC PLATELET DISORDERS

Autoimmune Thrombocytopenic Purpura

Pathophysiology. In autoimmune thrombocytopenic purpura platelets are coated with antibodies made by B lymphocytes. The platelets maintain their hemostatic function, but when the platelet passes into the spleen, with its surface altered by antibodies, the macrophages destroy the platelet. In the process, platelet antigens are then exposed to more B lymphocytes in the spleen and more antibodies are made by the spleenic lymphocytes. So, the spleen is not only the site of destruction of platelets, but also the site of antibody production, which then causes further destruction of platelets.

When plasma from clients with this disorder is infused into volunteers, the platelet count of the volunteer decreases rapidly and returns to normal in several days.

Clinical Presentations and Nursing Assessments. The client will have purpura on his arms, legs, upper chest, and neck. He will have mucosal bleeding. The disorder can be acute or chronic. The acute form is usually in children after viral infection, but it occurs in adults too without a preceding viral infection. There will be a sudden onset of bleeding, which is most severe initially. The risk of cerebral bleeding is greatest in the first 2 weeks. The client may display a bleeding tendency for several months, but most stop bleeding within the first 6 months. It can become a chronic state. When the client has recovered from the acute bleeding diathesis, he may have a compensated thrombocytolytic state where a near normal platelet level is maintained, but the client still has antibodies against his platelets. The client will make platelets at a slightly faster rate, and platelet survival is less than normal. These individuals should not be blood donors.

Laboratory Studies. The diagnosis is made by noting a decreased platelet count, large numbers of megakaryocytes in the bone marrow, antiplatelet antibodies, fever, and anemia. In the pregnant woman, the antiplatelet factor can be passed to the fetus, leading to a transient thrombocytopenia in the infant.

Medical Interventions. Most clients recover in time without treatment. Steroids can be used, which will interfere with phagocytosis of platelets in the spleen. They may also displace antibodies from platelets. For the refractory cases, splenectomy and immunosuppression are indicated. Nursing care is directed at caring for the bleeding client.

Thrombotic Thrombocytopenic Purpura

Pathophysiology. Thrombotic thrombocytopenic purpura (TTP) is a fulminating, usually lethal disorder, characterized by Coombs' negative hemolytic anemia with severely fragmented red blood cells, thrombocytopenic purpura, fever, renal failure, and fluctuating neurological manifestations. Many die within the first few weeks of onset of the disease. The cause is unknown. Platelets become sensitized, clump in blood vessels and plug them.

Clinical Presentations and Nursing Assessments. Diagnosis is made by noting the presence of severely fragmented red blood cells in peripheral blood. Hyaline thrombi are in the lumina of arterioles and capillaries, in the absence of vessel wall damage or inflammation. Blood coagulation values are normal, and platelet survival is decreased. Clinical manifestations are due to platelet thrombus formation, leading to multiple organ ischemic disease. For instance, the client may display strokelike symptoms as a result of thrombus formation in the brain.

Medical Interventions. Therapy is supportive. Large doses of prednisone with splenectomy is recommended, because the spleen may make antibodies. Penicillin in large doses is given to prevent platelets from clumping. Penicillin acts by coating platelet surfaces that blocks receptors to aggregating agents. Recently, plasma exchange in conjuction with antiplatelet agents, such as aspirin, has been used effectively. This approach may remove antibodies or immune complexes.

Nursing Interventions. Nursing care is that for the bleeding client. In addition, nursing measures directed at the specific consequences of thrombi is indicated. For instance, a client with strokelike symptoms may need nursing measures aimed at preventing complications of immobility. Mortality rate is 80 percent in the first 3 months, and 90 percent in the first year after diagnosis. The clients ultimately develop seizures, renal failure, and die.

VITAMIN K DISORDERS

Vitamin K disorders can be secondary to any condition that inhibits vitamin E absorption or intake. Vitamin K is not stored in the body and is a fat soluble vitamin essential for synthesis of prothrombin and factors VII, IX, and X.

A vitamin K deficiency can lead to a coagulopathy. Primary vitamin K deficiency is uncommon in healthy persons. This is due to widespread distribution of vitamin K in plant and animal tissues, and to the microbiological flora of the normal gut, which synthesize the substances that supply the bulk of the requirement for vitamin K. The causes of deficiencies in the vitamin K dependent coagulation factors are thus largely secondary to disease or drug therapy.

The causes in the adult are dietary inadequacies, total parenteral nutrition, biliary obstruction, malabsorption syndromes, liver disease, and drug therapy with coumarin anticoagulants, broad spectrum antibiotics, and megadoses of vitamin E.

Dietary Inadequacy

Foods that are high in vitamin K include broccoli, liver, egg yolks, and milk. Healthy adults fed on low vitamin K diets for several weeks show minimal signs of vitamin K deficiency unless they are given bowel-sterilizing antibiotics such a neomycin. Dietary deficiency becomes manifest much more quickly in debilitated clients with or without antibiotics.

Total Parenteral Nutrition

Physiological amounts of fat-soluble vitamins, particularly vitamins E and K, are not metabolized normally when introduced into the central venous circulation. It is advisable to administer vitamin E weekly to clients on prolonged total parenteral nutrition.

Biliary Obstruction

Obstructive jaundice and biliary fistulas can lead to impaired vitamin K absorption due to lack of bile salts. All clients with obstructive jaundice should receive parenteral vitamin K for 3 days prior to surgery.

Malabsorption Syndrome

Depression of the vitamin K-dependent coagulation factors is frequently found in the malabsorption syndromes and in other GI disorders, for instance cystic fibrosis, celiac disease, ulcerative colitis, and sprue. Such clients should be treated with all of the fat-soluble vitamins in doses that are about ten times the usual requirement (1 to 2 mg/day for vitamin K).

Liver Disease

Clients with parenchymal liver disease may have hypoprothrombinemia because of their inability to utilize vitamin K in the biosynthesis of vitamin K-dependent clotting factors. Vitamin K should be given along with other therapy for liver disease.

Coumarin: Drug-induced Hemorrhagic Disease

The coumarin anticoagulant drugs can induce serious hypoprothrombinemia. Some of the causes are reduction in dietary intake of vitamin K, ingestion of interfering drugs, and the inadvertent alteration of the anticoagulant dosage schedule. When overdosage accompanied by bleeding occurs, vitamin K is given parenterally until the bleeding is controlled (25 to 50 mg).

Broad-spectrum Antibiotics

An important source of vitamin K in humans is the intestinal flora. The GI bacteria may supply an individual's entire requirement. Vitamin K is not well absorbed from the colon, but most of the microorganisms synthesizing vitamin

K in the gut reside in the ileum. Sulfa drugs, neomycin, and other broad-spectrum antibiotics are capable of sterilizing the bowel. When a vitamin K deficient diet is provided, a serious bleeding tendency promptly develops.

Vitamin E

Large amounts of vitamin E may also antagonize the action of vitamin K.

Nursing responsibilities in vitamin K disorders include client teaching about foods high in vitamin K content and caring for a client with a bleeding disorder.

THROMBOCYTOSIS

Thrombocytosis is a platelet count of more than 1 million. It is usually temporary and may occur after severe hemorrhage, surgery, and splenectomy, in iron deficiency, and as a manifestation of occult neoplasm. It is associated with a tendency to thrombosis. Sustained elevation of a platelet count of more than 800,000 is called thrombocythemia and is a manifestation of one of the myeloproliferative disorders, for instance polycythemia or chronic lymphocytic leukemia (CLL). The client can have spontaneous bleeding secondary to leakage from damaged vessels, venous and arterial thrombosis, and necrosis of vessels distal to clots. Treatment is with anticoagulants.

BLOOD COAGULATION AND CANCER

It is a well known propensity of clients with certain forms of cancer to develop thromboembolic disease (TED) or DIC or both, commonly observed after rapid tumor lysis or surgical manipulation. The tendency for TED was first noted in 1865 by Armand Trouseau, who reported a high incidence of venous thrombosis in cancer patients. The overall incidence of clinical TED has been reported as 1 to 11 percent, but on postmortem examination, it is much higher. Thrombosis and bleeding is reported to be the second most common cause of death in hospitalized cancer clients. Clients particularly prone to TED are those with mucin secreting tumors of the GI tract, cancer of the lung, pancreatic cancer, and cancers of the colon and prostate. Clients with pancreatic cancer have the greatest risk of TED, with up to 50-fold increase in TED over controls with pancreatitis. These individuals are at an increased risk when treated with estrogen or chemotherapy.

Abnormalities of blood coagulation tests are found in 92 percent of clients with cancer. These abnormalities include an increased FSP level, thrombocytosis, and hyperfibrinogemia. It is theorized that low grade intravascular coagulation with accelerated clotting factor utilization is accompanied by an increased rate of synthesis for fibrinogen, clotting factors, and platelets. Occurrence of overt DIC is uncommon, but is seen with mucin secreting adenocarcinomas or predisposing conditions, for instance gram-negative sepsis or liver impairment. Overt DIC is seen in 9 to 15 percent of clients with cancer, but clinical DIC is common. Thrombocytopenia, abnormal platelet function, and evidence of in vivo activation of platelets have all been reported to occur with greater frequency in clients with cancer. Thrombocytosis occurs much more frequently in untreated clients with cancer. This may also be explained by the existence of low grade DIC, thrombocytolysia, and overcompensation. Qualitative abnormalities of platelet function have been described and may be secondary to increased FSP.

It is postulated that the interaction of tumor cells, platelets, and inflammatory cells may lead to the generation of a peritumor fibrin gel critical to the pathogenesis of tumor growth and metastasis formation. Although many investigators have suggested that fibrin acts as a glue, facilitating tumor cell adhesion to the endothelium, others maintain that tumor cells adhere independently to the endothelium, produce microinjury and secondary platelet adhesion with fibrin deposition. Even in the absence of endothelial injury, however, sequestration of fibrinogen and labeled platelets can be found at the sites of metastases of some animal tumors. Support for use of antiplatelet drugs and agents designed to produce thrombocytopenia in treatment of cancer derives from these experimental and clinical observations. Antiplatelet antibodies, capable of inducing thrombocytopenia, can significantly reduce the formation of lung implants following intravenous infusion of tumor cells in mice. This protective effect can be reversed with platelet transfusions. Drugs that impair platelet function have proved successful in treatment of cancer in experimental animals.

Inhibitory effects of anticoagulants on various properties of tumor cells have been recognized for at least 30 years. Coumarin derivatives can inhibit tumor cell locomotion, metabolism, lung colony formation, and development of spontaneous metastases in various experimental tumor systems. It appears that effects of coumarin drugs in treatment of cancer are mediated by their ability to interfere with the utilization of vitamin K. Experimental vitamin K deficiency provides similar protection from metastasis formation. Results of a Veterans Administration Cooperative Study on the use of warfarin in the treatment of small cell carcinoma of the lung—the first randomized controlled study of this agent as an anticancer drug—was recently published. Median survival of clients who received warfarin in addition to standard chemotherapy was significantly greater than median survival of subjects who received chemotherapy alone.

MANIPULATIONS OF THE COAGULATION SYSTEM

As discussed in other parts of this text, the coagulation system is being manipulated for treatment of various diseases. There is a great deal of research in areas other than disease treatment as well.

Progress in Thromboresistant Materials Research

Much research is being conducted on methods to improve thromboresistance of blood contacting materials, especially in the area of artificial substances— hemodialysis, artificial organs, cardiopulmonary bypass, and so forth. Prevention of thrombosis and embolization for a few hours in a high flow extracorporeal circuit is easily achieved in chronic hemodialysis or extracorporeal oxygenation by systemic anticoagulation and blood filtration. Even for such a short time, however, there is no doubt that microthrombi do form and that they do embolize. This is seen most critically in experiments with implanted small vessel grafts that set the most demanding standard for thromboresistance. Thromboresistance alone is an insufficient criterion for a blood compatible device. Susceptibility of other host defense mechanisms, for instance activation of immune mechanisms and inflammatory responses, and resistance to pathological responses, must be considered. In recent years, there has been a great deal of progress in the fundamental understanding of surface structures of polymeric implant materials, the mechanisms of contact activated coagulation, platelet adhesion and aggregation, and interactions of foreign materials with blood. Some particularly interesting work includes cultured endothelial linings, which confer patency and a stable lining on small artery grafts in dogs, and thromboresistant alkylderivatized polyurethanes.

Developers of these various approaches would be the first to state that there is, as yet, no perfect method for conferring thromboresistance on an arbitrarily selected implant material for an indefinite period of time. However, it is apparent from their collective work that substantial progress has been made toward this goal. Devices designed not only for blood contact, but also for exposure at other tissue sites, may well benefit from these techniques. This is important because we are entering an era of implantable device development that will provide artificial substances for almost all defective natural organs or segments of organs.

ANTICOAGULATION

Heparin

Heparin is the most familiar anticoagulant in use. It is derived either from pork intestine or beef lung. Because it is poorly absorbed from the GI tract, its exclusive use is parenteral.

Heparin works by accelerating the activity of antithrombin III. Antithrombin III is a circulating plasma protein, and neutralizes the activity of thrombin and other factors involved in the coagulation cascade. This inhibits further clotting by acting on prothrombin, factors V, IX, and X. When heparin is given prophylactically, its major effect is in inhibiting factor X, preventing the activation of prothrombin. It does not dissolve existent clots.

The activity of heparin is assessed by measuring the PTT, which is an assay of the intrinsic clotting system. The client's PTT is kept at 1½ to 2½ times that of the control.

A loading dose of 5000 to 10,000 units of heparin is given to achieve adequate blood levels, and is followed by an infusion rate of 1000 units per hour. This dosage is adjusted to maintain the PTT within its desired range. Heparin's half-life in the blood is about 90 minutes, therefore continuous infusion is the preferred method of administration. Prophylaxis against thromboembolism can be performed by giving heparin in minidose form. The drug is given subcutaneously to provide a gradual absorption of the drug. The effects of heparin are erratic with this method. They are maintained for about 6 to 8 hours. Bleeding can occur on heparin therapy, and the antidote for heparin is protamine sulfate.

Oral Anticoagulants

Available oral anticoagulants are derived from either coumarin or inandione. Primarily, coumarin derivatives are used clinically with warfarin sodium (Coumadin), the prototype.

Warfarin works by inhibiting the liver's activation of factors VII, IX, X, and II. Although the half-life of warfarin is moderate, the half-life of the clotting factors they inhibit is longer. Therefore, the activity of warfarin depends on the depletion of clotting factors, and effects are delayed accordingly.

Anticoagulation is achieved only when active circulating clotting factors have been depleted, requiring 6 to 8 days. For this reason, clients are started on warfarin while still on heparin. Effects are monitored by the PT, with the range being 1½ to 2½ times normal.

Bleeding can occur on oral anticoagulants, and the antidote is vitamin K. The therapeutic effect of warfarin can be increased by oral antidiabetic agents, chloral hydrate, clofibrate, salicylates, and sulfonamides. Other drugs that interact with warfarin in some way and place the patient at an increased risk of bleeding are: allopurinol, chloramphenicol, disulfiram, anabolic steroids, and thyroid preparations. Drugs that decrease the therapeutic effects are alcohol, barbiturates, carbamazepine, ethchlorvynol, glutethimide, rifampin, and estrogens.

CHAPTER 7

Alterations in Protective Mechanisms: Immune System Disorders—Decreased

No other area of physiology is as fascinating as that of the immune system. It is under intense scientific investigation as we begin to realize that the immune system controls or contributes to the functioning of every bodily process. Likewise, with a disorder of the immune system, every system of the body is affected. This has dramatic implications for nursing care.

Disorders of immunity due to hypoactive or insufficient functioning of the immune system can be either congenital or acquired. Immune deficiency disorders reflect an impairment in one or more of the major mechanisms of immunity. These are the physical defenses of the body, phagocytosis and bactericidal activity, inflammatory response, antibody responses, and cellular immunity responses.

Immunosuppression is a state of unresponsiveness of the immune system. The immune system cannot cope effectively with foreign antigens introduced into the body. Immunosuppression can occur to varying degrees, and can be a response to any number of events in the environment. Nursing and medical research has uncovered previously unknown etiologies of immunosuppression, including some that are within our therapeutic regimens. For instance, adverse environmental stimuli such as noise can lead to immune deficiency. In the typical intensive care unit, the noise level is very high. What implications might this have for the clients in that setting?

Immune system disorders present many exciting possibilities for nursing research. We can look at stimuli that may contribute to immunosuppression, for instance noise levels in the unit. Another area of research could be strategies for nursing care and demonstrating what are the optimal nursing measures for the immunosuppressed patient.

CONGENITAL IMMUNOSUPPRESSION

Congenital immunosuppression, or primary immune deficiency, are those diseases in which the individual is born with a failure of humoral antibody

TABLE 7-1. IMMUNOSUPPRESSION—ETIOLOGIES

Congenital Immunosuppression	Acquired Immunosuppression
B cell disorders	Age
Congenital hypogamma-	Nutritional status
globulinemia	Surgery and anesthesia
Selective IgA deficiency	Hospitalization
T cell disorders	Genetic defects
Di George syndrome	Adverse environmental events
Combined (T and B cell) disorders	Stress
Severe combined immunodeficiency	Psychiatric illness
disease (SCID)	CNS lesions

formation, a deficient cellular immune system, or a combined defect. The immune deficiency is not secondary to another condition (Tables 7-1 and 7-2).

B Cell Disorders

Congenital hypogammaglobulinemia

Clinical Presentation and Pathophysiology. The neonate is protected against infection by maternally acquired antibodies, specifically IgG. After the maternal immunoglobulins are no longer effective, at about 3 months of age, infants with this disorder experience repeated infections from bacterial organisms. They show no impairment in recovery from viral infections, for instance rubeola, rubella, mumps, or varicella. They are also not particularly susceptible to chronic superficial fungal infections. However, these babies do have a predisposition to autoimmune diseases.

The primary pathophysiology involved in congenital hypogammaglobulinemia is an absence of the mammalian equivalent of the bursa of Fabricus. The clients, therefore, lack B lymphocytes and their lymphoid tissues do not contain plasma cells.

TABLE 7-2. CONGENITAL IMMUNODEFICIENCY DISORDERS

Disorders	Lab Findings
B Cell	
X-linked	Reduced IgG ($\leq$ 200 mg/ul), absent IgM, IgA, IgD
hypogammaglobulinemia	IgE, absence of B cells in peripheral blood
Selective IgA deficiency	IgA $\leq$ 5 mg/dl
T Cell	
Di George's syndrome	Lymphopenia, absent T cell functions, ↓T cells
Combined	
SCID	Complete absence of both T and B cell immunity. Severe reduction or absence of T and B cells
Wiskott-Aldrich	Thrombocytopenia, normal IgG, ↓IgM, ↑IgA, ↑IgE.
syndrome	Inability to respond to polysaccharide antigens

Laboratory Studies. Diagnosis is made by immunoelectrophoresis, which shows deficiencies in one or more of the major immunoglobulin classes. Usually, the client has undetectable levels of IgM, IgA, IgE, and IgD. They produce essentially no antibodies to antigenic stimulation.

Medical and Nursing Interventions. Medical treatment consists of antibiotics whenever necessary, and injections of immune serum globulin to boost antibody levels. Nursing care revolves around goals and interventions for the care of the immunosuppressed (see Chap. 8).

Selective IgA Deficiency
Selective IgA deficiency is the most common of the primary deficiencies. The overall incidence is about 1 in 500. Many clients do not suffer from recurrent infections whereas others have repeated infections, autoimmune disorders, and increased risk of neoplasms. In those clients who are relatively asymptomatic, it is thought that other immunoglobulins compensate for the IgA deficiency. Clients who are symptomatic may have recurrent pneumonia, chronic bronchitis, sinusitis, chronic diarrhea, ulcerative colitis, or pernicious anemia. Allergies are common. It is speculated that the incidence of allergic symptoms may be due to an imbalance between secretory IgA and IgE, resulting in a competition for antigens. Transfusion reactions of the anaphylactoid type have also been reported.

Pathophysiology and Clinical Presentations. The pathophysiology behind the IgA deficiency is unknown. It is speculated that there may be an autoimmune component, because as many as 40 percent of IgA deficient clients have antibodies directed against IgA. Many of these clients have never received blood products where they could have developed these antibodies, and it is believed that they developed the antibodies from breast milk. Lymphocyte studies indicate that almost all affected individuals have IgA bearing B lymphocytes in their blood. Differentiation of these cells into IgA secreting plasma cells is blocked. A considerable body of evidence has accumulated indicating varying degrees of imparied T cell function.

IgA deficiency has been described in association with almost all of the major varieties of autoimmune disease, and the incidence in clients with systemic lupus erythematosus and rheumatoid arthritis seems to high to be coincidental (1 in 100).

Medical and Nursing Interventions. Diagnosis is made by noting the absence of IgA in respiratory secretions, serum, and external secretions. Treatment is supportive, consisting of antibiotics whenever an infection develops. Should blood transfusions be required, chance of a reaction can be minimized by freezing the client's own blood for future use, using donor blood from a matched IgA deficient person, or giving washed packed red cells.

Nursing care is directed toward caring for a client who is immunosuppressed (see Chap. 8). Teaching the client about his disease, signs and symptoms of infection, and the possibilities of allergic reactions and autoimmune disease is important.

T Cell Deficiencies

Di George's Syndrome

Pathophysiology and Clinical Presentations. The infant with Di George's Syndrome is born without his parathyroids or thymus. Therefore, he will suffer from neonatal hypocalcemia with tetany and cellular immunity defects. Other abnormalities commonly associated with this syndrome include low set, notched, or folded ears; hypertelorism; antimongoloid slant to the eyes; small, fishlike mouth; and abnormalities of the aortic arch and heart, including tetralogy of Fallot. Some autopsies have revealed a tiny, histologically normal thymus, usually in an abnormal location.

Immunological defects appear early in life usually within the first few months after birth. The infants will develop oral candidiasis, chronic diarrhea, failure to thrive, or chronic interstitial pneumonia. The overall health of the child is affected by the severity of the cardiovascular anomalies and the control of hypocalcemia.

Laboratory Studies. Diagnosis is made by noting lymphopenia, deficient numbers of E rosette forming T cells, deficient responses to antigens, cutaneous anergy, hypocalcemia, and hyperphosphatemia. Immunoglobulins and antibody responses are normal.

Medical and Nursing Interventions. Treatment options are limited. Under investigation currently are the use of thymic hormones or thymus transplants. Nursing care includes concepts appropriate to the care of the immunosuppressed (see Chap. 8). Support for the child's parents in dealing with this disease is essential and should include appropriate medication teaching and signs and symptoms of complications, especially those for hypocalcemia and cardiovascular problems.

COMBINED DISORDERS

Severe Combined Immunodeficiency

Pathophysiology. Among the inherited disorders, severe combined immunodeficiency represents the most severe form of immunological failure. It represents a group of disorders that have a variety of underlying lesions, occur in several genetic forms, and vary in the extent of immunological dysfunction. Combined immunodeficiency occurs in X-linked recessive, autosomal recessive, and sporadic forms. The disease may be due to a defect in the generation of lymphoid stem cells. This is supported by reports of successful reconstitution of immune functions with grafts of stem cells from fetal liver, and in some cases, from bone marrow. Recently, a considerable body of evidence has accumulated indicating that some forms of combined immunodeficiency may result from deficient thymus function.

Clinical Presentations. A neonate born with SCID manifests signs of recurrent infections, frequently with organisms of low pathogenicity within the first few months of life. These infections may be oral candidiasis, which can spread over the skin, pneumonias caused by viruses like cytomegalovirus, and opportunistic infections, for instance *Pneumocystis carinii*. They have chronic, resistant diarrhea, failure to thrive, and die within the first 2 years without appropriate treatment.

Laboratory Studies. Diagnosis is made by noting a marked reduction in lymphocyte counts. B and T lymphocytes are very few in number or absent from the peripheral blood and lymphoid tissues. Immunoglobulin levels are markedly reduced, except during the first 6 months of life as the infant will have maternally derived IgG. Peripheral blood lymphocytes fail to respond to antigens and antibody responses are feeble or nonexistent.

Antibody responses to polysaccharide antigens, for instance blood group substances, are weak. Thus, clients have low titers of isohemagglutinins. Cellular immune responses are abnormal also. There is a decrease in the absolute numbers of E rosette forming T cells. Cutaneous energy is common.

Medical Interventions. Treatment is to replace the missing component of the immune system. Transplantation of bone marrow or fetal liver from genotypically matched donors offers hope for patients with this disorder. Currently, thymus transplantation, especially the use of cultured thymic epithelium, injections of thymosin, and replacement of deficient enzymes is being evaluated.

Wiskott-Aldrich Syndrome

Pathophysiology and Clinical Presentations. The Wiskott-Aldrich syndrome is an X-linked disorder, characterized by thrombocytopenia, with a hemorrhagic tendency, eczema, and immunodeficiency with recurrent infections. The thrombocytopenia with bleeding tendencies appears during infancy. Eczema appears later. Infections involve the middle ear, and often lead to chronic otitis media. The clients are susceptible to infections from herpes viruses and lymphoreticular malignancies, especially of the central nervous system. The underlying mechanism is unknown. The defect may be at the level of the macrophage because of an inability to respond to polysaccharide antigens, but this is unconfirmed. Another factor that contributes to the low levels of immunoglobulins is hypercatabolism; there is evidence that the syndrome is characterized by a progressive depletion of immune responses. Young patients may have normal immunoglobulin levels but abnormalities appear with age.

Laboratory Studies. Male children with this disorder display thrombocytopenia, eczema, and recurrent otitis. The client has low levels of IgM, normal or increased levels of IgA and IgG, and extremely elevated levels of IgE.

Medical Interventions. The treatment is under investigation. The eczema responds to topical steroid therapy and local skin care. Severe thrombocytopenia may require platelet transfusions, but splenectomy is contraindicated because it may predispose the patient to sepsis. A few patients have received thymus grafts or bone marrow transplants, and in some cases, there have been definite and long lasting benefits. Transfer factor has been used in a number of clients with this syndrome, and somewhat greater than 50 percent of them have shown improvement in susceptibility to infections, chronic eczema, and reduction of splenomegaly. Most do not survive childhood, dying of complications of bleeding, infection, or lymphoreticular malignancy.

Nursing Interventions. Nursing care for children with SCID and Wiskott-Aldrich syndrome is complex. First, observe the procedures for nursing care of the immunosuppressed client (see Chap. 8). The parents of children affected with this disorder need much support. At the time of initial diagnosis, they may feel alone with their problems. A helpful support group, which the nurse can refer the parents to, is the Immune Deficiency Foundation (P.O. Box 586, Columbia, MD 21045). This foundation is a national voluntary health organization, set up by parents of children with immunodeficiency disorders. There are chapters throughout the United States and they will provide parents with information and access to individuals who are coping with similar problems.

When an immunodeficiency disorder is genetically determined, the parents must be provided with genetic counseling to help them comprehend the disease's transmission and the probability of having another child with the same disorder. In a few of these disorders, the parents and siblings of the client can be tested to determine if they are carriers of the disease. Amniocentesis may be performed to determine if a fetus is affected. All of these considerations and options must be explained and brought to the attention of the parents. Psychological support should be provided to these parents who may be overwhelmed with guilt or depression from learning that the illness is inherited.

In many instance, the parents of a child with an immunodeficiency disease must accept and deal with the fact that their child has a chronic or potentially fatal illness. In these cases, the nurse plays a key role in helping families deal with the stress of overwhelming illness, impending death, or threat of death. Nurses can help by using referrals to services such as visiting nurse associations for help with the physical aspects of care, and parents' groups and clergymen for help with the psychosocial aspects of the illness. Nurses can also assist families by providing information to school teachers and administrators or by establishing contact with community agencies that provide financial assistance.

Generalizations About T and B Lymphocyte Deficiencies

Deficiencies in B cell function lead to deficiencies in antibody formation or humoral immunity. The individual will have infections due to encapsulated bacteria. These organisms infect people who have normal B cell function also, but only when neutropenia or a complement deficiency is present. This suggests that a collaboration involving antibodies, complement proteins, and phagocytes exist as the chief mechanism of defense against pyogenic organisms. Agammaglobulinemic (without antibodies) individuals, who have normal cellular immune system function, have an interesting response to viral infections. The clinical course of primary infection with viruses does not differ significantly from that of the normal host. However, long lasting immunity may not develop and as a result, multiple bouts of chickenpox and measles may occur. Such observations suggest that T cells may be sufficient for control of the established viral infections whereas antibodies play an important role in limiting the initial dissemination of the virus and in providing long lasting protection. Exceptions to this generalization are becoming widely recognized. For instance, agammaglobulinemic clients fail to clear hepatitis B from their circulation, and have a progressive, and often fatal course.

Deficiencies in T cell function lead to deficiencies in cellular immunity. Cellular immune defects lead to overwhelming infections with organisms such as *Candida*, cytomegalovirus, pneumocystis, disseminated herpes, and other opportunistic bacteria, viruses, and fungi. T cell deficiency is probably always accompanied by some abnormality of antibody responses, although this may not be reflected by hypogammaglobulinemia. This may explain in part why clients with primary T cell disorders are also subject to overwhelming bacterial infections. Attenuated live virus or bacterial vaccines can produce fatal infections. Blood transfusions can cause graft versus host reactions and should be given only under controlled circumstances, or for therapy of the immune deficiency state. Even then, the blood must be irradiated before administration to destroy leukocytes.

ACQUIRED IMMUNODEFICIENCY STATES

Acquired immunodeficiency states are associated with an underlying pathologic state. Immune deficiencies occur often during the course of many acute and chronic diseases. Virtually any severely ill person may have compromised immune defenses.

Age influences immune function. Immune function is depressed in the very young and the elderly. Of the population over 80 years of age, 63 percent are estimated to be anergic. This fact has dramatic implications for nursing because a majority of elderly people are incapable of generating an immune response to an antigen. This explains why elderly clients become infected so readily after being admitted to a hospital. They cannot fight off pathogens.

A client's nutritional status has a major impact on immune functioning. Protein and caloric malnutrition can alter immune responses and resistance to infection. Protein and calorie malnutrition leads to a diminished ability to form circulating antibodies, defects in antigen processing and recognition, and diminished phagocytic abilities. In the adult, lymphatic tissues atrophy. Impaired cellular immunity is evident by all standard tests. Protein-energy starved patients experience a higher incidence of morbidity and mortality during common infections than well nourished individuals, and are subject to opportunistic infections. Impaired respiratory function is a common cause of death. Protein malnutrition and iron deficiency result in atrophy of liver, spleen, bone marrow, and lymphoid tissues.

Malnutrition seems to alter certain aspects of the humoral immune system as well. Most malnourished individuals are reported to have a decreased antibody response to certain antigens, especially yellow fever, flu, and typhoid vaccines. Additional effects of protein and calorie malnutrition on the immune system include a reduction in the secretory antibody response in the respiratory, gastrointestinal (GI), and genitourinary tracts. These effects, coupled with atrophic mucosal barriers, can easily increase the host's susceptibility to invasions by organisms covering these mucosal surfaces.

Malnutrition may interfere with recovery from infectious diseases. For example, the walling off processes initiated by an infecting agent requires the synthesis of fibrin, polysaccharides, and collagen. In a malnourished client, these responses are retarded because of an inadequate intake of essential precursors, including protein.

Surgery and anesthesia affect immune system functioning. Both B cell and T cell capabilities are inhibited by halothane, cyclopropane, ether, and nitrous oxide. Anesthetic agents depress allergic responses and inhibit phagocytosis. Although these studies are based on limited samples, a generalization can be made that postoperative clients have deficient immune system functioning.

When a client is hospitalized, there is a slow conversion of his original flora to a flora more reflective of the hospital's organisms. The longer a client stays in the hospital prior to surgery, the greater his chance of a postoperative wound infection. Similarly, the longer the operation, the greater the risk of infection.

Some genetic defects are associated with acquired immunodeficiency states. The genetic defects that affect the susceptibility or resistance to infection include sickle cell anemia, G6PD deficiency, and many hemoglobinopathies. Genetic susceptibility is correlated with racial and sex factors. This is reflected in the increased incidence of tuberculosis in nonwhites. Furthermore, a greater proportion of male rather than female infants suffer from serious bacterial infections. Recently a relationship has been demonstrated between histocompatibility types and susceptibility to certain infectious diseases.

There is evidence to suggest that adverse environmental events can have a significant influence on susceptibility to infection, growth of tumors, and immunologic function in animals. High intensity sound, shock avoidance, or repeated exposure to a predator can increase susceptibility to infection with certain viruses in mice. Similar adverse stimuli protects monkeys, however, against infection. Therefore, when monkeys are exposed to adverse stimuli, they are more capable of resisting infections than those monkeys who are left alone. Perhaps this research can be generalized to humans. Maybe a little stress or adverse events in our lives helps us to fight infection. Future research may hold the answers. Animals administered shock avoidance have a decreased susceptibility to polio virus. Daily handling of mice decreases survival time after inoculation with leukemia virus. There are many studies such as these that have repeatedly shown that environmental events can influence the expression of clinical disease. However, many of these studies lack reliability and validity, and the results have often been contradictory from system to system. This particular area of research is a fascinating one, with great potential for application of human life-styles. Further progress in this area necessitates the development of precise methodologies, but the possibilities are enormous. How does a hospital environment, particularly an intensive care unit, affect the client's immune system? One could speculate that an intensive care unit is an adverse environment, and based on the early research done in this area of science, is potentially immunosuppressive.

There have been many studies looking at the relationship between stressful life events and subsequent development of disease. One of the earliest studies was done by two investigators, Holmes and Rahe. They studied the relationship between life events in humans and the onset of illness, using a tool known as a Social Readjustment Rating Scale and Schedule of Recent Events. This scale assigned values to each of 43 life events such as birth, marriage, divorce, or death of a spouse, based on the change that each of the events caused in the individual's pattern of life. The study reported a positive, linear relationship between the quantity of life change units accumulated in one year, the likelihood of illness onset, and the severity of illness. These correlations were statistically significant but low, accounting for only a small proportion of the variance of illness onset. This study was important because it initiated an entirely new area of inquiry. Methodologically, however, the study was weak because it was very broad and because of its low correlations.

Other studies have looked at widows and widowers in their period of bereavement. One group followed widows and widowers, and a control group, for a period of 14 months. The bereaved group had more physical and psychiatric illnesses than the control group. They also showed lymphocyte abnormalities 8 weeks, but not 2 weeks, after bereavement.

A host of other stressful situations have been studied in relation to their effects on the immune system. One study looked at the effects of 72 hours of sleep deprivation on the phagocytic abilities of the individual. Results showed an increase in interferon level, a decrease in phagocytosis, and a decrease in lymphocyte reactivity. It is unclear from this early study how much of an immunosuppressive effect sleep deprivation has on an individual. Further research is necessary, but it does pose an interesting question. Are nurses who rotate shifts frequently subject to more infections than their stable shift colleagues?

The study of specific stressful events, such as bereavement or sleep deprivation, offers experimental control and the possibility of studying interviewing variables. Studies such as these are rapidly expanding our data base and generating new questions and possibilities for nursing research.

Psychiatric illness has been associated with immunological abnormalities. Investigators have reported that schizophrenic clients show some signs of immunosuppression. They show a normal reactivity to purified protein derivative (PPD) injections but a decreased wheal response to histamine. They have impaired lymphocyte responses. Rheumatoid factor, a sign of autoimmune disease, has been found in the serum of schizophrenics. One study reported that two to three times as many psychiatric versus general medical clients, or normal blood donors, had anti-brain antibodies in their serum. When this serum was injected into monkeys, the animals had electroencephalogram and behavioral changes.

Rheumatoid factor has also been associated with endogenous depression. All of these studies did not control the effects of endogenous glucocorticosteroids or demonstrate any consistent effects of psychiatric illness on the immune system.

Several investigators studied the effect of central nervous system (CNS) lesions or CNS stimulation on the immune system. The results of these experiments suggest that lesions of the CNS, especially of the hypothalamus, produce changes in the immune response and in some cases the histology of lymphatic tissues. However, it is difficult to compare the studies because the investigators have lesioned different parts of the CNS and measured different immune responses. In addition, there is not a large enough body of data with one animal system to draw final conclusions about the role of the CNS.

Many investigators over the last 60 years have described attempts to change the immune response through behavioral conditioning. Much of this work has centered around immunosuppressing mice with cyclophosphamide, paired with saccharin for conditioning purposes. Subsequent exposure to saccharin elicited immunosuppressive responses similar to those produced by cyclophosphamide. Repeated reports of statistically significant conditioning of the immune response suggests that the phenomena is real. However, the actual experimental change is relatively small and is not uniform in every subject. These investigations were well designed and these data do suggest that the potential of the brain to modulate immunological reactivity should be examined in greater detail.

To summarize, there are many factors that can influence or hamper a client's immune system. These factors, many of which have only been investigated within the last 3 years, are separate and distinct from "therapeutic" immunosuppression, induced by chemotherapy, radiotherapy, steroids, and other drugs.

THERAPEUTIC IMMUNOSUPPRESSION

Drugs

Immunosuppression with drugs is defined as a negative control or regulation of immunological reactivity. There are several major categories of immunosuppessive drugs: cytotoxic agents, corticosteroids, and antilymphocyte globulins which is discussed in greater detail with bone marrow transplants.

Cytotoxic Drugs
Chemotherapeutic agents or cytotoxic drugs are used not only for the treatment of neoplasms but for other immunologically mediated diseases as well. Because the pathogenesis of many of the immunologically mediated diseases that are treated with cytotoxic agents is unclear, it is difficult to delineate the precise mechanisms whereby cytotoxic agents cause clinical improvement in a particular disease. It is possible that clones of aberrantly reactive lymphoid cells are selectively eliminated by the drug. In a less specific manner, the general antiinflammatory and immunosuppressive effects may control the abnormal immune reactivity until the stimulus is removed or until a state of tolerance ensues naturally.

Chemotherapeutic agents work during the cell cycle. The cell cycle is a process of replication. Rate of cell replication varies with each cell type. Some cells, like neurons, are highly differentiated and have lost their capacity to divide. Other cells have a short life span and are in a constant state of renewal, for instance, blood cells, hair follicles, and epithelial cells of the GI tract. Phases of cell activity within the cycle are indicated by G_0, G_1, S, G_2, and M. G refers to gap and designates the time interval gaps between synthesis of DNA(S) and mitosis(M). G_0 is the resting phase, and cells can remain in this phase for varying lengths of time. They are capable of entering G_1 when activated or at times of increased demand. G_1 is the stage when cells are preparing for DNA synthesis. Synthesis of RNA and protein is ongoing. In G_2, synthesis of RNA continues. In the S phase, DNA is synthesized. In the M phase, the cell splits into two daughter cells that contain the same number and kind of chromosomes as the parent cell. They can then either mature and replicate, or enter G_0 and await activation.

Chemotherapeutic drugs exert their effects at the cellular level by interfering with the cell cycle. Although antineoplastic drugs cannot distinguish

108

TABLE 7-3. ANTINEOPLASTIC DRUGS—USAGE

Drug	Use	Comments
Alkylating Agents		
Busulfan (Myleran)	Chronic myelocytic leukemia (CML)	BMD, N + V Irreversible pulmonary fibrosis (dose-related) hyperuricemia
Chlorambucil (Leukeran)	Chronic lymphotic leukemia (CLL), Hodgkin's disease, ovarian cancer	BMD, N + V
Cyclophosphamide (Cytoxan)	Breast lymphomas, ovarian, lung	BMD N + V, alopecia, mucositis/stomatitis, hemorrhagic cystitis
Mechlorethamine (nitrogen mustard)	Hodgkin's disease	BMD N + V, mucositis/ stomatitis, alopecia
L-Phenylalanine mustard (Alkeran)	Breast, ovary, multiple myeloma	BMD, N + V
Triethylene- Thiophosphoramide (Thio-Tepa)	Ovary, breast, lymphoma, bladder	BMD, N + V
Antimetabolites		
Cytosine arabinoside (Ara-c)	AML	BMD, mucositis, stomatitis, N + V, diarrhea, hepatotoxicity
5-Fluorouracil (5FU)	Breast, ovary, colon, gastric	BMD, N + V, alopecia, mucositis, stomatitis, hepatotoxicity
6-Mercaptopurine (6MP)	ALL, AML	BMD, N + V, mucositis, stomatitis, hepatotoxicity
Methotrexate (MTX)	Breast, ALL, meningeal leukemia, head and neck, lung, osteogenic sarcoma, chorio carcinoma	BMD, mucositis, stomatitis, GI ulceration, diarrhea, hepatotoxicity, nephrotoxicity, CNS toxicity with intrathecal
6-Thioguanine (6TG)	AML	BMD, N + V, diarrhea, hepatotoxicity
Antitumor Antibiotics		
Bleomycin	Testicular, lymphoma, head and neck, cervix	Fever, myalgia, pulmonary fibrosis
Dactinomycin (Actinomycin-D)	Ewing's sarcoma, rhabdomyosarcoma, Wilms' tumor	BMD, N + V, mucositis, stomatitis, diarrhea
Daunomycin	AML	BMD, N + V, mucositis, stomatitis, alopecia, cardiac damage

TABLE 7-3. (Cont.)

Drug	Use	Comments
Doxorubicin (Adriamycin)	AML, breast	BMD, N + V, mucositis, stomatitis, diarrhea, alopecia, red urine, dose related cardiomyopathy
Mithramycin	Breast, cervix, pancreas, gastric	BMD, N + V, mucositis, stomatitis, alopecia
Nitrosoureas		
2-Chlorethyl nitrosourea (BCNU)	CNS tumors, multiple multiple myeloma	BMD, N + V ⎫ Cross blood– brain
3-Cyclohexyl nitrosourea (CCNU)	Hodgkin's disease, CNS tumors, GT, lung	BMD, N + V ⎭ barrier
Vinca Alkaloids		
Vinblastine (Velban)	Hodgkin's disease, testicular	BMD, N + V, neurotoxicity
Vincristine (Oncovin)	ALL, Wilms' tumor, soft tissue sarcoma	NV, alopecia, neurotoxicity
Miscellaneous		
DTIC	Malignant melanoma, Hodgkin's disease	BMD, flu-like syndrome, hepatotoxicity
Cis-Platinum	Testicular, ovarian	BMD, NV, neurotoxicity, nephrotoxicity
Procarbazine	Hodgkin's disease, lymphoma	BMD, NV, peripheral, neuropathy, Mao inhibitor
Hormones		
Diethylstilbesterol (DES) Estinyl	Breast	N + V, fluid retention, changes in libido, uterine bleeding, nipple discoloration, hypercalcemia
Megace provera	Uterine, breast, renal cell	
Halotestin	Breast	N + V, fluid retention
Steroids	Many	Na^+ and fluid retention, electrolyte imbalances, hypertension, osteoporosis, muscle weakness, GI bleeding, menstrual irregularity, latent diabetes mellitus, acne, psychosis, moon face, lymphocytes

BMD = Bone marrow depression, N + V = Nausea + vomiting.
Note: Not a complete listing of drugs, side effects, toxicities, or administration. Reader should consult pharmacology literature for more information.

between normal and malignant cells, normal cells can repair themselves more readily and effectively than cancer cells.

Antineoplastic agents are classified according to their chemical structure and function at the cellular level. Alkylating agents cause cross linking and abnormal base pairings of protein and interfere with DNA replication. Antimetabolites exert their effect during synthesis of DNA by inhibiting synthesis of protein, or by deceiving the cell by inserting the wrong metabolites. Antitumor antibiotics inhibit RNA synthesis. Hormones interfere with the synthesis of protein and alter cell metabolism by changing the cell's hormonal environment (Table 7–3).

Chemotherapeutic agents may be used singly or in combination with other cytotoxic drugs and treatment (radiation therapy, immunotherapy, surgery) for the curative or palliative treatment of many types of cancer. In recent years, adjuvant chemotherapy—the use of antineoplastic drugs to enhance the patient's response to other forms of cancer therapy—has proved useful in prolonging life and, in some instances, of curing certain types of cancer. The goal is to destroy residual micrometastatic disease after primary cancer therapy, usually surgery, has been employed. It has proved particularly useful in treatment of Wilms' tumor, testicular cancer, osteogenic sarcoma, Ewing's sarcoma, and Hodgkin's disease.

Cytotoxic agents, particularly cyclophosphamide at extremely high doses, have been shown to have profound effects on practically every aspect of cellular and humoral immune responses. Different cytotoxic agents have been shown to suppress all parameters of immune reactivity. In the treatment of immunologically mediated diseases, cytotoxic agents are almost always administered to suppress an ongoing immunological process. Low to moderate doses are usually administered for a prolonged period of time. It is felt that the major mechanism of immunosuppression of these agents is quantitative of absolute lymphocytopenia. Cytotoxic agents are used in rheumatoid arthritis, systemic lupus erythematous, membranous glomerulonephritis, chronic active hepatitis, inflammatory bowel disease, autoimmune hemolytic anemia, immune thrombocytopenia, and others. The major immunological effect is on the lymphocytes that have been stimulated to differentiate by antigen, as well as killing unstimulated lymphocytes. Usually, these drugs do not act on antibody-producing cells.

There are long-term complications of cytotoxic therapy. They include susceptibility to infections by opportunistic organisms, for instance *Pneumocystis carinii* and increased risk of cancer; renal transplant clients have a hundred times greater chance of developing cancer, usually lymphomas, than a control group of the same age.

The nursing care required by the individual on chemotherapy is complex and multifaceted. Many of these drugs lead to bone marrow depression. The client will, therefore, be quite prone to infection, due to granulocytopenia, and bleeding, due to thrombocytopenia. The nursing care for these two situations is discussed elsewhere in this text. Many drugs cause mucositis and stoma-

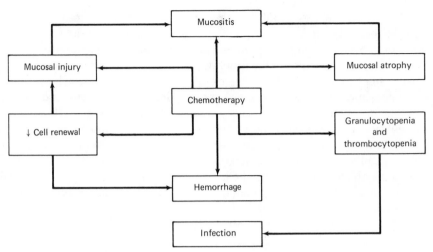

Figure 7-1. Effects of chemotherapy in the mouth.

titis of the oropharynx, and can involve the esophagus. The ulceration secondary to chemotherapy, as well as a decreased amount of saliva is painful to the client, and can greatly inhibit adequate nutritional intake. An effective therapeutic regimen for stomatitis involves mouth sprays with a solution of normal saline, peroxide, and sodium bicarbonate, effective pain control with a topical agent, and thorough dental hygiene. Ice chips and popsicles can be helpful as a comfort measure. Many clients suffer from nausea and vomiting from the chemotherapy. Use of antiemetics should be encouraged. Small, frequent meals are often tolerated better than three large ones. Alopecia is a frequent side effect of many drugs. Scalp hypothermia, although not consistently effective, has been shown to be helpful for doxorubicin hydrochloride-induced alopecia in doses of 50 mg or less. Therefore, it may be offered to anyone except those with leukemia. The scalp can be a storage site of leukemic cells. Micrometastases can lodge in scalp tissue. By using hypothermia, chemotherapeutic agents will not reach the scalp. These micrometastases can lead to relapse at a later date. The client on a chemotherapy program needs tremendous support from the nurse. Teaching about drug effects, prevention of infection, possible drug toxicities, and self-care are just a few aspects that need to be included in the nursing care plan. The client needs emotional support about the many changes in body image and alterations in life-style due to chemotherapy (Fig. 7-1 and Chap. 8).

Steroids

It has frequently been said that, if you do not know what else to do, give steroids. Although their beneficial effects are often dramatic and their efficacy has been clearly established in several diseases, the hazards and side effects of these agents are numerous and must always be considered when embarking on therapeutic regimens.

Steroids achieve their anti-inflammatory effects through stabilization of vascular beds. Leakage of fluid and cells into inflammatory sites is thereby decreased. Steroids decrease granulocyte and monocyte accumulation in inflammatory sites and inhibit the functions of these cells. Steroids also suppress various steps in the immediate hypersensitivity reaction. They achieve their immunosuppressive effects by decreasing circulating lymphocytes and monocytes; by decreasing certain lymphocyte and particularly monocyte functional capabilities; and by decreasing immunoglobulin and complement levels.

Following a single large dose of steroids, there is a prompt reduction in blood lymphocytes, reaching a maximum after 4 to 6 hours. The number of T cells is reduced significantly, the number of B cells is decreased to a lesser extent. This leads to a lymphopenia, due to a redistribution of lymphocytes in the body, not due to lymphocyte destruction. The lymphocyte count returns to normal within 24 hours after administration of steroids. Of interest is the fact that, at the point of maximal lymphocytopenia, there is very little, if any, suppression of the functional capabilities of the lymphocytes left in the circulation. Therefore, one of the major effects of steroids on lymphoid cells, in doses commonly used in inflammatory and immunological diseases, is not a qualitative functional suppression but a quantitative depletion of lymphocytes from the circulation, thus making them less readily available to the tissue involved in the immunological reaction. There also appears to be a lower limit of lymphocytopenia beneath which even massive doses of steroids cannot push the lymphocyte count. In fact, the degree and kinetics of lymphocytopenia that follows a wide range of doses of steroids, from approximately 20 mg of prednisone to as high as 1 g of methylprednisolone, are strikingly similar. There is a temporary increase in the number of circulating neutrophils, resulting from an increased release of cells from the bone marrow, and a demargination of those cells adherent to the endothelium of blood vessels. A decrease in the marginal pool of leukocytes thereby reduces the ability of the host to respond to inflammatory stimuli, as their presence in the marginal pool and the potential capability of leaving the vascular compartment are diminished. This prevents the accumulation of neutrophils at inflammatory sites—the primary anti-inflammatory reaction. There is a striking decrease in the number of monocytes and eosinophils, and there is an inhibition of the functional activity of these cells, which limits their ability to participate in immune and inflammatory functions.

Steroids, when administered over a long time, result in a modest decrease in serum immunoglobulin concentrations with serum IgG more affected than IgA and IgM. Human volunteers given 96 mg of methylprednisolone daily for 3 to 5 days had a 22 percent decrease in IgG as compared to controls. Cellular responses are also inhibited by steroids. Clients taking steroids may manifest an inability to express cutaneous hypersensitivity responses (anergy) despite previous sensitization. The impaired cellular immunity seen in clients on long-term steroid therapy may result from several different effects of steroids on the immune system, including inhibition of migration of T cells to the site of antigen deposition; inhibition of lymphokine release from lymphocytes; decrease in monocyte numbers; and blocking interaction between lymphocytes and monocytes.

Corticosteroids cause a depletion of cells from the intravascular recirculating pool of lymphocytes. The depletion is caused by a redistribution of cells, out of the circulation, from the intravascular to the extravascular recirculating pool. This causes a depletion in the intravascular space of predominantly long lived T cells, part of a total body recirculating pool of cells that under normal circumstances have relatively free access into and out of the intravascular space.

In vitro steroids have been shown to suppress phagocytosis and microbicidal functions of neutrophils. When used in suprapharmacologic concentrations they stabilize granulocyte lysosomal membranes and decrease inflammatory responses by blocking the release of lysosomal enzymes. In addition, the responses of granulocytes to chemotactic factors are suppressed by high concentrations of in vitro steroids. However, it appears that the major neutrophil-related effect of steroids at pharmacological in vivo concentrations is a blockage of cells from reaching the inflammatory site, with a relative sparing of actual functional capabilities.

To summarize, steroids display the following immunological effects (Table 7-4):

1. An anti-inflammatory action by decreasing the number of cells available to participate in the inflammatory response, stabilizing vascular beds, and reduction of the functional capabilities of immunologically active cells.
2. Temporary lymphocytopenia due to redistribution of lymphocytes from the intravascular to the extravascular recirculating pool.
3. Temporary increase in neutrophils and decrease in monocytes and eosinophils.
4. With chronic administration, decrease in immunoglobulin concentrations and cellular immune system functioning.
5. Suppression of functions of neutrophils, monocytes, and eosinophils.

The side effects are numerous. They include increased susceptibility to infections, cushingoid body, cataracts, glaucoma, diabetes mellitus, osteo-

TABLE 7-4. IMMUNOLOGICAL EFFECTS OF STEROIDS

1. Anti-inflammatory
2. Lymphocytopenia—temporary
3. Temporary increase in neutrophils
4. Decrease in monocytes and eosinophils
5. Chronic steroids—decrease in immunoglobulin concentration and cellular immune system functioning
6. Suppression of functions of neutrophils, monocytes, and eosinophils

TABLE 7-5. SIDE EFFECTS OF STEROIDS

1. ↑ Susceptibility to infections	10. Suppression of hypothalmic–pituitary–adrenal axis
2. Cushingoid body	
3. Cataracts	11. Retardation of growth in children
4. Glaucoma	12. Aseptic necrosis of bone
5. Diabetes mellitus	13. Pancreatitis
6. Osteoporosis	14. Intracranial hypertension
7. Psychological disorders	15. Poor wound healing
8. Hypertension	16. Peptic ulcers
9. Electrolyte disturbances	17. Hypercatabolism

porosis, psychological disorders, hypertension, electrolyte disturbances, suppression of the hypothalamic–pituitary–adrenal axis, growth retardation in children, aseptic necrosis of bone, pancreatitis, intracranial hypertension, poor wound healing, exacerbation of peptic ulcers, and hypercatabolism (Table 7–5).

The most effective immunosuppressive regimen, namely high dose/divided dose daily therapy, is associated with the most severe side effects. If the total dosage of the drug is lowered, and as one goes from a single daily dose to an alternate day dose, there are relatively few side effects. With alternate day steroid regimens, for the entire off day and part of the on day, monocyte and lymphocyte counts, proportions of lymphocyte subpopulations, various functional capabilities of cells, and all other measurable parameters are normal. Such regimens are quite effective, in certain diseases, in maintaining a state of remission, despite the fact that inflammatory and immunological reactivity are normal for at least half the time.

In summary, corticosteroids have the potential to directly suppress the functional capability of lymphocytes and monocytes or interfere with their availability to the immunological reaction, or both. Certain monocyte functions are quite sensitive to steroids. From a practical standpoint, most of the lymphocyte functional capabilities, for instance mediator production and release, cytotoxic effector activity, and even proliferative responses, are relatively resistant to pharmacologically attainable concentrations of steroids. It should be mentioned that although immunoglobulin production in humans can be suppressed somewhat by high doses of steroids, specific antibody production, particularly in secondary IgG responses, is quite resistant to steroid therapy. Thus, it appears that the major mechanism whereby pharmacological concentration of steroids exert their effects on lymphoid cells is by interfering with their availability to the immunological reaction.

Other Drugs Causing Immunosuppression
Other drugs that cause immunosuppression by inhibiting cellular immunity are: tetracycline, chloramphenicol, clindamycin, streptomycin, gentamycin,

kanamycin, and neomycin. Mafenide and silver sulfadiazine (Silvadene) can inhibit chemotaxis by polymorphonuclear neutrophils.

Because we have a good foundation in the multiple etiologies of immunosuppression, we can now look at two of the most commonly encountered categories—AIDS and transplants.

ACQUIRED IMMUNE DEFICIENCY SYNDROME

Epidemiology

Since 1981, acquired immune deficiency syndrome (AIDS) has become a major health problem in this country. It has reached epidemic proportions in major metropolitan areas. In the summer of 1981, the Centers for Disease Control (CDC) announced to the health care community an outbreak of 25 cases of *Pneumocystis carinii* pneumonia and Kaposi's sarcoma in homosexual men who were clustered in New York City and California. By March of 1982, 300 cases had been reported. As of January 1985, 8000 cases have been reported. Forty-seven percent of those cases have died. No one has been cured. In 3 years time, at the present rate of infection, AIDS will claim 100,000 people, and in 5 years time, 1.6 million. The people at risk are homosexual or bisexual males (71 percent) intravenous drug abusers (17 percent), Haitian immigrants (5 percent) hemophiliacs (1 percent), and a "miscellaneous" group, some of whom have received blood transfusions in the past, others who have been female sexual partners of bisexual men, and children born to parents who are in risk groups for AIDS. (6 percent). The disease has primarily affected men. The women involved have been intravenous drug abusers or sexual partners of bisexual men.

Currently, the mortality rate is 40 percent. However, more than 70 percent of the clients with the earliest diagnosed cases have died, which predicts that the ultimate mortality will be approximately 85 percent.

According to one study by the CDC, homosexual or bisexual clients report a very active sexual life-style—1100 contacts in one lifetime, whereas a control group reports approximately 500 contacts. Ninety-eight percent of clients report a history of exposure to nitrites. However, the history of nitrite usage is just as prevalent in a control population, with approximately 85 percent of healthy male homosexuals in New York and California reporting its use. Use of nitrites is closely correlated with numbers of sexual partners, and with specific homosexual practices, social events, and meeting places. Amyl nitrite and other drugs are sold legally under such names as "Rush," and are used as sexual stimulants.

Pathophysiology. There is much speculation about the etiology of AIDS. The immune dysfunction is believed to have an infectious basis. Among homosexuals, sexual transmission is almost a certainty. Through exhaustive case tracking, CDC researchers were able to trace sexual encounters between 40 patients in 10 different cities. Mapping these sexual histories revealed an incubation pattern, the time between infection and onset of symptoms, of a few months to more than 2 years. Epidemiologists believe that it can be spread via sexual contacts and blood products, and other means of transmission may yet be identified.

The degree of immunodeficiency that develops is extraordinary, and not approached even in clients treated chronically with cyclosporin A and cyclophosphamide. Kaposi's sarcoma and opportunistic infections appear to be secondary to the acquired immune dysfunctions. Clients with autoimmune disorders and renal transplants have an increased incidence of Kaposi's sarcoma. When immunosuppressive drugs are discontinued, the sarcoma lesions can regress, suggesting that immunodeficiency is primary, and malignancy and infections are secondary.

Kaposi's sarcoma was initially described in 1872, in Vienna. It typically occurs in men, with an average age of 63, and more frequently in men of Italian and Jewish descent. Typically, it has an indolent course, and is seldom fatal even 5 to 10 years after diagnosis. The dark blue or purple brown plaques occur usually on the lower extremities, and are responsive to chemotherapy. The Kaposi's sarcoma seen in AIDS clients, however, is affecting young men, and has an aggressive course that can lead to lymphadenopathy, visceral lymph node involvement, and tumors in internal organs. Lesions occur on the face and upper extremities, and the mean survival time is 15 months. The etiology of Kaposi's sarcoma is unknown, but the fact that it is endemic in certain areas suggests genetic, infectious, or environmental factors. Cytomegalovirus (CMV) infections have been suspected because CMV can produce degrees of immunosuppression. Antibody titers to CMV are higher in Kaposi's sarcoma clients compared to control. In addition, CMV DNA and gene products can be found in tissue samples of about one-third of the sarcoma patients.

Because of the high incidence of Kaposi's sarcoma and the nature of opportunistic infections, defects in cellular immunity are felt to be the pathogenesis in AIDS. Humoral immunity is normal with normal or increased levels of antibodies. The client will have low lymphocyte counts, often less than half of the normal range. T lymphocytes are decreased in number and abnormal in composition, whereas B lymphocytes are not impaired. The helper T cell population is decreased, or even absent, whereas killer T cells are normal or increased in number. Loss of the helper cells with an intact killer subpopulation suppresses cellular immunity, and allows opportunistic infections to develop.

Although the defect in host defenses is broad, the infections developing in AIDS clients are primarily those associated with defective cellular immunity, the so-called opportunistic infections. An opportunistic infection develops only in individuals who lack normal immune defenses. The organisms are typically ubiquitous in nature, and are not particularly virulent to the immune competent individual. Clients who suffer from the various types of immunosuppression, particularly of the cellular immune system, become infected and ill from these same organisms. They include CMV, *P. carinii*, herpes, *Candida*, and *Cryptococcus*. The clients most susceptible to opportunistic infections are those receiving chemotherapy and radiotherapy, and those with other acquired immunodeficiency states, such as AIDS.

Etiology. CMV, a form of herpes virus, may play a role in the development of AIDS. It can be transmitted sexually via the urine and the semen and is virtually endemic in the homosexual male population. The virus can persist in the semen at a high titer for months. Following a CMV infection, very high titers of the virus can be shed in the semen of asymptomatic subjects for more than a year. It is likely that sexually active homosexual men are frequently reinfected through exposure to semen and urine of their sexual partners. Although CMV can cause mild immunosuppression in animals, to date it has not been associated definitively with Kaposi's sarcoma or opportunistic infections. CMV has been recovered from secretions in most of AIDS patients, and significant increases in antibody titers indicate recent infection or reactivation. Because more than 90 percent of the homosexual males have antibodies indicating previous CMV infections, positive cultures can merely represent reactivation of latent infection during immunosuppression as happens in transplant patients. There is no evidence that primary CMV infections is more common in patients with this new syndrome than in matched homosexual controls.

Human T cell leukemia virus (HTLV) is the etiological agent in AIDS. It is a retrovirus that was first described in 1980 in a patient with mycosis fungoides. It is known to cause leukemias, lymphomas, and solid tumors in several species of animals and T cell malignancies in humans. It also causes immune deficiency in some cats infected with feline leukemia virus. The mechanisms by which HTLV is transmitted is unknown. Transmission by blood transfusion is probable. The rate of infection in spouses of patients with T cell lymphoma is elevated, therefore HTLV may be transmitted by sexual or other intimate contact. The virus is endemic in southern Japan and the Caribbean. Evidence of exposure to HTLV has been found in 25 to 40 percent of AIDS clients. Isolation of virus, viral DNA in T cells, and a much higher incidence of antibodies against HTLV in the AIDS clients than in controls have all been found. This is significant. The prevalence rate for exposure to HTLV was at least 10 to 40-fold higher in the AIDS clients than in homosexual controls, a situation not seen for other infectious agents evaluated in the same individuals.

The target cell for AIDS is the T cell. Because HTLV is a T cell retrovirus, it can be linked hypothetically to other human T cell disorders. The finding of AIDS in Haitians who may not have been exposed to other risk factors for the disease may be important because HTLV is endemic in the West Indies.

Clinical Presentations and Nursing Assessments. The client initially seeks health care for a variety of symptoms and signs such as diarrhea, loss of weight, malaise, fever, and frequent infections. Physical assessment reveals wasting, lymphadenopathy, fever, and possibly Kaposi's sarcoma lesions. The disease course is variable. AIDS has a broad spectrum of events beginning with an asymptomatic acquired immune abnormality, or latent period. The client is infectious to his sexual partners at this time although being entirely asymptomatic. The latent period can last up to 2 years. This is followed by a prodromal period, with fever of unknown origin, diarrhea, weight loss, malaise, lymphadenopathy, and wasting. Opportunistic infections and Kaposi's sarcoma may then develop. Infections described include viruses, bacteria, fungi, and protozoa. Death occurs as a result of the opportunistic infections.

Laboratory Studies. Laboratory evidence of cellular immunity dysfunction demonstrates lymphocyte abnormalities. The client has cutaneous anergy. Anergy, a state of unresponsiveness of the immune system, is demonstrated by the lack of response to various antigens injected subcutaneously. He will have profound lymphopenia, especially of the T lymphocyte population, decreased lymphocyte proliferation responses, defective natural killer cell activity, and a deficiency in interferon.

Medical Interventions. The treatment is supportive. Many clients are on prophylactic trimethoprim for *P. carinii.* Other drug agents being evaluated include interferon, interleukin 2, and transfer factor. One client had a bone marrow transplant facilitated because he had an identical twin, but this was unsuccessful in changing the course of the disease.

Nursing Interventions. The psychosocial consequences of the disease are enormous. There has been an increasing amount of public hysteria, which has spread, in part, to the health care community. The homosexual community is finding itself ostracized and feared as a possible source of disease. It cannot be denied that some of the basis for this reaction is of a discriminatory and homophobic nature, as the disease cannot be spread through casual contact. It is the responsibility of the health care professional to dispel myths and hysteria among lay people through education regarding the limited infectivity of the disease, and appropriate preventative measures. The CDC has recommended that, while hospitalized, the AIDS client be placed on blood and body fluid precautions.

TRANSPLANTATION

One modality of treatment for immunologically mediated diseases is bone marrow transplantation. Marrow transplantation is a rational therapeutic option only if the client's disease involves the bone marrow, or if hazard to the normal marrow is the limiting factor in the aggressive treatment of a disease. A marrow transplant involves a transplant of donor hematopoietic system, lymphoid and macrophage system. It is used for three primary conditions:

1. Immunological deficiency disease—Marrow grafting is used to replace the individual's genetically deficient immune system with the donor's normal lymphoid system. An example is use of the bone marrow transplant in the treatment of SCID.
2. Aplastic anemia—This disease process results in loss of marrow, and transplantation is done to replace the client's defective organ with a normal one.
3. Leukemia—The client's leukemic cell population and normal marrow cells are destroyed by intensive chemoradiotherapy and is replaced by the transplanted, normal marrow.

Marrow transplantation is conceptually different from transplantation of other organs, for instance a liver. The only thing asked of a transplanted liver is that enough of it survives in the recipient to provide adequate liver function. With marrow, a tiny fraction of the organ is asked to regrow to a normal size and then keep on growing for the rest of the person's life. In addition, the allogenic marrow transplant carries lymphocytes that recognize the host as foreign and can induce fatal graft versus host disease. Rather than conceptualizing this procedure as an organ transplant for the recipient, it may be thought of as a "body" transplant for the marrow cells.

There are three types of marrow transplants:

1. Autologous—Marrow is taken from an individual, stored, and reinfused after the client has received a very large dose of cytotoxic therapy for various cancers.
2. Syngeneic—Marrow from an identical twin, or a genetically identical individual.
3. Allogeneic—Donor and recipient are different genetic origins. This is the most complex because measures must be taken to avoid graft versus host disease.

Procedure

Each family member donates blood for testing. A suitable donor is selected, and possible donors for granulocytes and platelets can be identified. This is done by determining histocompatibility or the human leukocyte antigen (HLA) type. The HLA type refers to a group of antigenic substances found on many cells types, including white blood cells and platelets. The HLA complex is composed of a series of genetic loci on chromosome 6. There are two major loci and two minor loci. The array of antigens encoded by this region on one chromosome is known as a haplotype. Each individual has two haplotypes, one inherited from each parent. Within a family there can be only four haplotypes. Each sibling has one chance in four of being HLA identical with the patient. The most preferable transplants are those between HLA identical siblings because they are the most compatible form of allogenic transplants.

The number of different antigens that exist in the population is large. Over 20 antigens have been identified in each major locus and all of them are fairly common. So, there are literally thousands of possible combination for the four antigen composition of a given individual determining his HLA type.

An identical twin constitutes a special example of an HLA identical sibling who is matched not only for HLA, but for all genetic loci. Although only a small fraction of clients will have an identical twin, these transplants have been very effective therapeutically and scientifically informative because the twin provides marrow that is like the client's own, except that it is free of disease.

Generally, there is no natural immunity to HLA antigens. Sensitization usually occurs through pregnancy or through exposure to platelets and white blood cells in past transfusions. Unsensitized persons may receive platelets from unmatched donors with good results for a time. Eventually repeated transfusions of random platelets will lead to diffuse sensitivity to common HLA antigens not present in the recipient. In individuals so sensitized, additional random platelets will not raise the platelet count and may cause transfusion reactions. This can be a catastrophic problem in the posttransplant period.

Despite tissue typing, there continues to be problems during marrow transplantation associated with reactivity in histocompatibility antigens other than HLA that cannot be identified at this time. These will manifest themselves as graft versus host disease and graft rejection.

A donor is chosen who shares with the recipient all or part of the major histocompatibility complex. Red blood cell incompatibility is not a barrier to marrow transplantation.

After HLA typing has been completed, the donor is taken to the operating room where multiple aspirations are done to retrieve bone marrow. The only restriction is that the donor be in good general health. Approximately 100 to 150 aspirations are performed to obtain 500 to 800 cc of marrow. The aspirations are from the sternum, pelvic bones, and ribs, primarily. As each aspiration is performed, the marrow is mixed with heparin and tissue culture medium. When the collection is completed, the marrow is passed through stainless steel screens to break up marrow particles. It is then transferred to a blood transfusion bag.

The client, meanwhile, has had a Hickman double lumen catheter inserted. This is a silicone catheter placed into the sublavian vein. A 4-inch subcutaneous tunnel is made in the chest and the catheter is threaded from an exit site above the client's nipple to the initial incision site at the neck. A small Dacron cuff is attached to the catheter and lies in the tunnel to provide a barrier to the migration of microorganisms. Connective tissue will grow around the cuffs, and acts as an anchor for the catheter. The catheter makes it possible to administer hyperalimentation, medications, and blood products, and is also used for drawing blood samples. About 90 percent of clients have the catheter in place for approximately 3 months. Other catheter alternatives include the double lumen Hickman/Broviac catheters.

The leukemic clients are prepared with large doses of cyclophosphamide and total body irradiation, to totally destroy leukemic cells and the host's immune system to allow engraftment. Clients with aplastic anemia receive cyclophosphamide alone, and infants with SCID are conditioned to accept a transplant by the nature of their disease.

The marrow is administered to the client by intravenous infusion into the Hickman catheter. The marrow stem cells pass through the lungs, and subsequent growth and reconstitution of the marrow is confined almost exclusively to the medullary cavity. In other words, it is administered through the Hickman catheter and migrates to the places where it can grow best. The infusion is usually given over 4 hours, and the client may experience chills, fevers, and hives. These effects can be minimized by the administration of small doses of meperidine intravenously, or diphenhydramine. If the client has a diminished cardiac reserve, he may show signs of fluid overload. This complication must be closely watched for, as well as for the possibility of micropulmonary emboli.

The posttransplant period is very difficult and complicated. The client is without any immunity whatsoever for a minimum of 10 days. It takes 10 to 20 days before the donor stem cells begin to proliferate and mature. This is a critical period, and supportive care is essential for survival. The primary problems in this period are infection, bleeding, nutrition and hydration, and psychosocial adaptation.

Currently, under investigation is a technique of mixing marrow with a soybean protein that isolates mature lymphocytes so that they can be removed. Remaining immature lymphocytes can theoretically be given to the client because these cells will acquire tolerance to his tissues and function normally.

Complications

Potential for Infection
Because the client is without immunity for 10 to 20 days, the chances of infection are great. Prophylactic broad-spectrum antibiotics may be given, especially if the client becomes febrile. Granulocyte transfusions may be given in this period of marked granulocytopenia, or when there is a documented sepsis. These transfusions are irradiated with 1500 rads prior to infusion to destroy the killer T cells and prevent a transfusion reaction. Nursing care of the immunosuppressed client is vitally important and will be discussed at length in Chapter 8.

Potential for Injury Related to Bleeding
The client will have low platelet counts, and therefore may demonstrate petechiae, epistaxis, mouth and gastrointestional bleeding, and conjunctiva and

cerebral hemorrhage. Platelet transfusions from compatible donors are often needed to maintain platelet counts above 20,000. Hematocrits are maintained with transfusions to maximize the oxygen carrying capacity of the blood. The nurse caring for this client should institute bleeding precautions (see Chap. 5).

Potential Alteration in Nutritional Status

The client must have a high protein, high calorie diet to redevelop his immune system. In addition, when malnutrition is combined with the stresses of transplantation, the chances of morbidity and mortality may increase. Total parenteral nutrition, consisting of amino acids, vitamins, minerals, carbohydrates, and fats, is administered. Effectiveness of this therapy should be determined by a dietitian. Fluid and electrolyte status is monitored closely to correct any problems quickly.

Potential for Ineffective Coping

This period of time is enormously stressful for the client. He has many stressors imposed upon him within a short period of time. Foremost of these is that the client is confronted with a life threatening disease. Additionally, other major stressors, including changes in body image and self-concept, a sense of loss, and forced dependency affect the behavioral responses of the client to his illness. An essential component in the recovery of this client is his relationship with his nurse. A bone marrow transplant necessitates a long hospitalization. The client will be very sick for most of his inpatient time and is constantly made aware of the gravity of his condition and the many potential life threatening complications. He will be called upon again and again to cope with these stressors. The client can follow one of two avenues. He can *react* to each new stress as he has in the past, becoming increasingly anxious and possibly resorting to a hostile or withdrawn behavior. The other avenue is that the client, with his nurse's active support, anticipate stressors and utilize new coping mechanisms which he had not realized he possessed. With a supportive nurse–client relationship, this can be a growth experience for both parties involved.

Graft Versus Host Disease

Graft versus host disease (GVHD) is a major problem in the transplant patient. It results from new circulating, competent donor T cells that immunologically attack host tissue. Virtually all cells in the body have different determinants for histocompatibility but manifestations of GVHD are essentially linked to the skin, liver, and gastrointestinal tract.

Infusion of nonirradiated blood products can also cause this syndrome in immunologically compromised patients. Therefore, all blood products given to the transplant recipient are irradiated. This inhibits proliferation of lymphocytes while leaving intact platelets, white blood cells, and red blood cells.

GVHD is acutely present in 30 to 60 percent of transplant recipients, 15 percent of whom die. One study reported a series of 262 clients given a marrow graft from an HLA identical sibling, all of whom received prophylactic treatment against GVHD, and yet 44 percent developed moderate to severe GVHD.

A skin rash is usually the first sign of GVHD and may progress to generalized erythroderma and desquamation. Liver involvement may manifest itself in the form of elevated enzymes, icterus, or ascites. Gastrointestinal signs include cramps, diarrhea—which may be profuse—and melena. Severe immunological deficiency accompanies GVHD, and death from infection is often the terminal event.

The treatment is preventative by the use of immunosuppressive therapy. Cyclophosphamide and methotrexate have been used. However, clinical trials of these regimens are not yet conclusive. Antithymocyte globulin (ATG) is an antiserum made of immunoglobulin fractions of serum from horses, goats, and rabbits immunized by injections of human lymphoid cells. It is used in cases of clinically established GVHD, and improvement has been noted in some individuals. It may contain high titers of antibodies against specific subsets of T cells. Other modalities of treatment for this problem are currently under investigation. They include steroid therapy, cyclosporin A, and monoclonal antibodies. The recent development of monoclonal antibodies that react with human T cells or subsets of T cells, points the way to greatly improved methods of in vitro treatment of marrow. Cyclosporin A is a fungal metabolite and an extremely potent immunosuppressive agent. It has been found to be without significant marrow toxicities and has a preferential effect upon early activation of helper T cells, thereby augmenting suppressor T cell responses. Assessment of this agent is currently under way in a number of trials, but early results are encouraging. It seems to work well only in conjunction with corticosteroids. Some incidence of nephrotoxicity, hepatoxicity, and lymphomas has been reported.

Other Complications

Late Infections
The transplant client has pronounced immunologic impairment for up to 4 months following the procedure, and it is 12 to 18 months before he regains a normal immune system. As a result, the client is prone to developing infections.

Interstitial pneumonia occurs in at least 40 percent of clients surviving 30 days posttransplant. The fatality rate is high, approximately 60 percent. Half of these pneumonias are due to CMV, the other cases are primarily due to idiopathic causes. The prophylactic use of interferon and CMV immunoglobulin parenterally for CMV is being studied, because there is no effective treatment for this infection at present. There is little doubt that the intensive chemoradiotherapy these clients undergo predispose them to pneumonia. *P. carinii* has been almost eliminated since the widespread use of trimethoprim and sulfamethoxazole for the prevention and treatment of this opportunistic protozoa. Herpes zoster or the varicella virus is a late infection that is common also.

Venoocclusive Disease
Venoocclusive disease is a disease of the liver occurring in 20 percent of clients. It usually occurs in the first 3 weeks posttransplant, and results from fibrous obliteration of the hepatic circulation. The signs include hepatomegaly, ascites, hepatocellular necrosis, and encephalopathy. It can be fatal.

Marrow Graft Rejection
In the case of rejection, the marrow graft functions for a while, and then fails. The peripheral blood counts suddenly drop and marrow biopsy shows the marrow to be devoid of myeloid elements. It is usually a consequence of sensitization of the recipient by transfusions against antigens present in the donor. Inadequate immunosuppressive therapy before grafting may facilitate marrow graft rejection. It is a common problem in clients with aplastic anemia, but is rare in leukemic clients.

Chronic Graft Versus Host Disease
Chronic graft versus host disease is a complication in about 30 percent of transplant recipients who survive beyond 100 days. It may be mild to severe. Manifestations include skin disease, severe oral and esophageal mucositis, malabsorption, pulmonary insufficiency, chronic liver disease, recurrent bacterial infections, and generalized wasting. One treatment for this complication currently under investigation includes prednisone and either procarbazine, cyclophosphamide, or azathioprine.

Recovery

After a period of profound granulocytopenia, engraftment is usually signaled by a rise in granulocytes and platelets, and the reappearance of reticulocytes. The median time required to reach a granulocyte count of 100/per cu mm is 16 days, and to reach 1000/per cu mm is 26 days. The rise in platelet counts usually lags a week or two behind the rise in granulocyte counts. Proof of engraftment depends on the use of cytogenetics and blood genetic markers to confirm that regenerating marrow is of donor origin. The client can go home when his white blood count is above 500 per cu mm, when he is eating more than 1000 calories per day, and when there are no signs of infection. The marrow will be composed of the donor's myeloid system, lymphoid system, and monocyte/macrophage system.

The bone marrow transplant is an extremely complicated procedure. The ethical problems of exposing a client and a donor to the marrow transplant regimen have limited its use. However, the demonstration of better long-term survival with marrow transplantation compared to conventional therapy for younger clients with severe aplastic anemia or acute leukemia should mitigate the ethical concern.

ALTERNATIVE WAYS TO INCREASE IMMUNITY

Immunotherapy

Immunotherapy is being used currently for treatment of various types of cancer. There are three types of immunotherapy: active, passive, and nonspecific. Active immunotherapy is using specific cancer antigens to stimulate specific host immune responses. Passive immunotherapy is the use of antibodies, sensitized cells, or immune RNA or transfer factor made outside the host. Nonspecific immunotherapy is the use of various noncancer antigens to stimulate the immune system nonspecifically.

Nonspecific immunotherapy is most commonly used at present as an experimental, therapeutic technique with some effect in some clients. Attenuated live bovine TB bacillus (BCG), is used as a nonspecific stimuli for the reticuloendothelial system. It improves humoral and cell-mediated immunity. It activates macrophages. In clients with melanoma and other cancers, it gathers lymphocytes to sites of tumor nodules. It is given via scarification, intralesional, intracavitary, intravesical, intrapulmonary, intradermally, or orally. Side effects include allergic reactions. Another agent used for immunotherapy is dinitrochlorobenzene (DNCB).

Interleukin

Interleukin is a lymphokine of which there are two types. Interleukin II is a T cell growth factor, and is being used clinically in that way. The isolation of specific T cell growth factors is changing the approach to understanding T cell function. This class of growth factors has allowed the establishment of a number of T cell lines. Because interleukin II is a growth factor for T cell clones, it provides an ability to isolate T cell clones of different phenotypes and should allow immunologists to detail the cellular interactions required to generate different immune responses. Both interleukin I and II stimulate antigen dependent, cell-mediated, and humoral immune responses. Interleukin II only can stimulate continuous growth of T cells. It is being used clinically in defects of cellular immunity—cancer, AIDS, and others.

Monoclonal Antibodies

Monoclonal antibodies are antibodies directed against a specific antigen. Clinically they are being used against tumor cells. They are pure homogeneous antibodies of defined specificity and are being used as "antibody therapy." Studies show that leukemia cells can be cleared from the blood temporarily. B cell malignancies present a special opportunity to test the potential of antibody therapy. Each B cell tumor expresses a unique cell surface IgG common to all members of the malignant clone and different from all normal B cells of the host. The idiotype of tumor cell surface IgG represents the closest approximation of tumor-specific antigen available. Nonsecreting B cell malignancies are perfect candidates for anti-idiotype therapy because they are not associated with high serum levels of idiotype protein that could block the effects of the antibody. Diseases in this category are follicular lymphoma, Burkitt's lymphoma, and chronic lymphocytic leukemia. Reports on its use are limited.

Interferon

Interferon acts by initiating DNA directed RNA synthesis and protein synthesis. Possibly messenger RNA (mRNA) is translated and yields a protein that has an antiviral effect. Interferon inhibits viral nucleic acid or viral proteins. It inhibits DNA synthesis in cells and may activate or suppress certain components of the immune system. Rate of growth of a new protein molecule is depressed by interferon. Its antitumor effects are thought to act by inhibiting tumor virus replication, cell transformation by virus, and inhibition of tumor growth through effects of the immune system. It has been noted to inhibit allograft rejection, graft versus host disease, delayed hypersensitivity reaction, and tumor cells. It is being used for a number of malignancies, with some reports of tumor regression. Side effects include fever, nausea, vomiting, chills, lassitude, erythematous skin reactions, and with larger doses, mild bone marrow depression. Other uses include vericella, herpes zoster, chronic hepatitis B, osteogenic sarcoma, and AIDS.

CHAPTER 8
Nursing Care of the Immunosuppressed Client

An immunosuppressed client is one who has a diminished, or even absent, ability to respond to an immunological challenge. This client depends on his nursing care for coordination of all aspects of the therapeutic regimen, to protect him from infection, to be cognizant of the functioning of all body systems, and perhaps most importantly, to be cared for in a holistic, humanistic way. The care of the immunosuppressed client is very complex. However, these clients are exciting to care for, because nursing care often makes a dramatic difference in their recovery and rehabilitation.

ASSESSMENT

History. Obtain a history of the current illness from the client. Information about prior hospitalizations and the client's reactions to his treatment and health care providers may supply important data for the formulation of a plan of care. Elicit information about the client's prior coping patterns. He may cope by overeating, drinking, "talking it out," or exercise. What is his family or significant other's reaction to his illness?

Nursing Assessments. Nursing assessment of this client, on a frequent basis, is vital. A systems approach allows for comprehensive data gathering. By utilizing the same steps in the assessment process with each client, the nurse is less likely to overlook clinically important findings. A systematic approach to nursing assessment includes evaluating subjective and objective data concerning each physiological body system, psychological dimensions, social factors, spiritual dimensions, and responses to illness and therapy.

During assessment, the nurse needs to be extremely attentive to possible sites of infection in these clients. Note any signs of local inflammation or systemic infection, changes in temperature, and changes in laboratory findings, particularly the white blood cell count and differential. Recognition of infection in neutropenic clients is often difficult. Fever may be the only sign because the classic signs and symptoms of inflammation—pain, redness, swelling, or heat—may be diminished or absent due to the absence of neutrophils, the first line of defense.

Observe closely intravenous sites, infection sites, and pressure points for any signs of impending infection. Perianal infections are frequent in immunosuppressed clients, and the nurse should closely observe all such body crevices. Absence or paucity of lymph nodes, in an infected area, is an important physical finding to note. Careful auscultation for adventitious sounds in the chest should be performed frequently. Evaluate the client's general affect and appearance in nutritional status plays a key role in immune system functioning.

Nursing Interventions. For the immunosuppressed client, nursing interventions will be directed at the prevention of infection, the maintenance or improvement of nutritional status, and psychosocial needs.

ALTERED PROTECTIVE MECHANISMS: LEUKOPENIA

Infection is a major cause of morbidity and mortality in the immunosuppressed client. Septicemia is a common sequelae of bacterial, parasitic, viral, and fungal infections. Sepsis is a life threatening condition, and the goal of much of nursing care is to prevent it. Extreme care should be used in all nursing procedures for the immunocompromised individual. Frequent thorough handwashing is imperative. Unrelenting aseptic technique in the care of all possible entrance sites for infection is vital. These sites include all catheters, central lines, endotracheal tubes, pressure monitoring lines, and peripheral intravenous lines. Nursing care assignments should be made with attention to the possibility of cross-contamination. Care should be delivered first to the immunologically depressed client to avoid this problem.

Statistics show that infection in the immunosuppressed client is derived from endogenous flora. In other words, the client becomes infected from organisms normally inhabiting his body. Additionally, organisms that are ubiquitous in the environment are virulent to these clients. Ubiquitous organisms include *Pneumocystis carinii*, cytomegalovirus, and acinetobacter. The procedure of reverse isolation is highly controversial in the immunosuppressed client, namely because it cannot prevent the endogenous and ubiquitous organisms from causing infection. Studies show that neutropenic clients have the same incidence of infection whether they are cared for in reverse isolation or in a private room. Precautions that must be taken when the client is cared for in a private room are:

1. Strict, frequent, thorough handwashing.

2. Masks for all persons with upper respiratory infections who must enter the room.
3. Masks for both client and nurse when a central line is entered.
4. Private room with the door closed to minimize cross-contamination.

Other precautions that need to be observed are: damp dusting, with a disinfectant solution, of the objects in the client's room every 24 hours; humidification of the air to reduce microorganisms that thrive in arid environments; and constant vigilance against standing collections of water where microorganisms can breed, especially vases, denture cups, suction containers, and respiratory therapy equipment. Any standing collections of water, which must be in the client's room, should be changed at least every 24 hours.

Skin care is very important in the immunocompromised host. The skin is the only intact defense that many of these clients have, therefore the nurse should be observing all possible pressure areas closely for signs of infection or breakdown. Turning is necessary every hour, if the client is immobile. Passive or active exercises for joints is important, as is avoidance of prolonged contact with wetness, which macerates skin. The skin should be well lubricated as dry skin can crack and allow antigens into the circulation.

Pulmonary toilette should be performed every 4 to 6 hours. Many of the opportunistic organisms lead to a pneumonia. Frequent assessments and coughing, deep breathing, and postural drainage are vital for prophylaxis and early detection of an infection.

A person with an immunological disorder should not receive immunization with a live virus such as oral polio, measles, or rubella, or should their siblings or other household contacts. The administration of live viruses to someone who is immunosuppressed can result in serious illness or death.

POTENTIAL ALTERATIONS IN ORAL MUCOUS MEMBRANES

Clients who have received chemotherapy or radiotherapy are likely to develop stomatitis. This is problematic for two reasons. First, it presents a likely source for infection. Second, it impairs the client from eating a diet high in protein and calories, essential factors for a normal immune system.

Assess the client daily for signs and symptoms of stomatitis: edema, increased temperature sensitivity, pain or burning, ulcerations, lesions, and color changes such as erythema and pallor. Observe for any white, opaque lesions that could indicate candidiasis. Interventions that may prevent oral infection from developing in a client with stomatitis are to brush the teeth with a soft toothbrush or toothette and use a mild nonabrasive toothpaste such as Crest or Sensodyne. Have the client rinse his mouth with saline every 4 hours. Avoid commercial mouth washes, and hot, spicy foods that irritate an already inflamed mucosa. If an infection does develop, the client will receive appropriate antibiotics.

ALTERATIONS IN NUTRITION: LESS THAN BODY REQUIREMENTS

To redevelop his immune system, the client must have a high protein, high calorie diet. When malnutrition is combined with the stresses of immunosuppression, the chances of morbidity and mortality increase. Total parenteral nutrition, consisting of amino acids, vitamins, minerals, carbohydrates, and fats, is given if the client cannot maintain an adequate diet by mouth. Effectiveness of this therapy should be determined weekly by a dietitian. Fluid and electrolyte status is monitored closely to correct any problems quickly.

POTENTIAL FOR INEFFECTIVE COPING

The client with an immunodeficiency disorder has many stressors imposed on him within a short period of time. He is faced with a life threatening disease, numerous hospitalizations, life threatening therapy, changes in body image, changes in self-concept, a sense of loss, forced dependency, and changes in role. All of these stressors can affect the behavioral responses of the client to his illness.

Self-concept includes such aspects as body image and role, and is subject to continuous development from stimuli in the environment and significant others. Once the self-concept has been formed, it serves as a frame of reference for reality, and all experiences are interpreted in terms of it. Body image, as an entity, is derived from past and current experiences; it is the way we see ourselves. Illness alters the self-concept and body image by interrupting the normal life situations and perceptions of self. For instance, the individual's perceptions of his state of well-being, his physical integrity, and his abilities to be independent and self-sufficient are changed. Threats to self-esteem, identity, role, and sexual identification may ensue.

Many medical and nursing activities—bone marrow transplantation and use of life-sustaining equipment and intrusive procedures—force the individual to realize how critically ill he is, and so alters his concept of self. Concurrently, the patient experiences feelings of sadness or loss over what has been lost or changed—his independence or his role as provider, for instance. His sense of totality as a human being is lost and a grieving process often will ensue.

Forced dependency, or loss of control, is a significant stressor for critically ill clients. His life and future are in jeopardy and he is unsure of the outcome of his illness. The environment of the hospital is a source of stress because it is grossly unfamiliar to the client and is filled with complex and unfamiliar equipment. The client is exposed to multiple stimuli from various sources and is confined in a small space, with monitor leads and tubes attached. He has lost control over his activities of daily living—eating, sleeping, elimination, attire, and activity levels. His privacy is invaded at random, and others decide whom and when he visits, what and when diagnostic tests are performed, who performs them, and what treatment he receives.

Normally, levels of control in daily life are incorporated into one's identity. Upon admittance to an intensive care unit or marrow transplant unit, the client becomes totally dependent upon unknown persons and mysterious machines for his survival. He is forced into a dependent role in which he must be cared for and remain relatively passive. The crisis that is precipitated by an illness necessitating marrow transplant, for instance, suddenly alters all aspects of his functioning. The client's physical capabilities and control over his personal life, interpersonal relations and mobility are affected, and his power to carry on self-imposed goals and obligations is lost. This role change from a self-sufficient, independent individual to one who is helpless, sick, and restricted can lead to frustration, fear, and ultimately, intense anxiety. This anxiety within the client may be behaviorally manifested as hostility and anger. Some clients have expressed the view that these feelings of lack of control and helplessness can seem more menacing than the threat of death.

Because the client is a passive, rather than an active, participant in his care, he is subject to a strong, regressive force. He is put into bed and infantalized with surrogate parents who pay constant attention to him and minister to all his needs. Physical pain and low energy levels, depressed awareness from drugs and hypoxia, sensory overload from high noise levels and constant disturbance, loss of time orientation from perceptual daytime lighting and sleep deprivation, and constant movement of people can create an almost frantic feeling of lack of control and anxiety.

Sensory deprivation is a particularly acute problem in this client population. Many hospitals employ reverse isolation, or the even more severe marrow transplant unit, for the bone marrow transplant patient or immunodepressed client. The lack of physical contact and feelings of isolation can precipitate acute loneliness, hallucinations, sleep disorders, and behavioral disorders. This environment fosters depersonalization. The client is an object being treated, a person having things done to him or for him, divested of his human capacities and functions.

The nurse caring for a client in this situation can continually assess the psychological impact of the illness and hospital environment on the client, his family, and the staff, and employ appropriate nursing measures to lessen anxiety and enhance comfort. However, rather than dealing with each behavioral response by matching a particular nursing intervention, a holistic approach requires the nurse to get to know the client well enough to ascertain why a particular response has been manifested. Our heightened awareness of the client as a psychobiological unit, our acceptance of the important of holism in the management of the critically ill client, and our planning and implementation of nursing interventions that incorporate all aspects of the person can greatly enhance the quality of our nursing care. Such an approach can help ensure that the client's psychological response to his disease does not impair his ability to return to full functioning.

Although many clients can cope with their disease and the effects of treatment, there are those who are not able to overcome their vulnerability. This can vary in its manifestations, duration, and intensity. It has been said that the client's vulnerability is an index of the distress he is experiencing. It may range from feelings of helplessness to resentment, from anxiety to loneliness. The impact of the client's disease and treatment is felt by his family and other members of the support system. However, it is primarily the family who offers support and who realizes significant disruptions in almost every area. The client's and his family's ability to adapt depends on the resources available within the family and the larger support system. These resources are influenced by the family's previous experiences, adaptability, and ability to integrate change, their social and economic status, and the support of the extended family and community.

Social support systems can help to ameliorate the effects of a crisis and assist the individual to cope with its impact. Family, friends, and other clients may provide an effective support group throughout the course of disease.

How can we incorpoate aspects of all systems of a client into his care to enhance his control over the situation? First, we can recognize that while the presence of a critical illness necessitates the use of various procedures and equipment that will interfere with the client's sense of self, we can work around this obstacle. By remaining cognizant of the client's uniqueness—his strengths, weaknesses, life-style, goals, character traits, aspirations, and previous experiences—we can support the particular coping mechanism that helps him deal with his illness and the necessary therapeutic interventions. As we make this psychological assessment, in conjunction with a physiological assessment, we help to reassure the client that someone cares about him and his reaction to illness. The client's family or significant others should be included in this assessment, as they are an integral system interacting with the client.

There are many ways in which we can incorporate the individuality of the patient into his care and lessen his feelings of dependency. In doing so we can be more creative than, for example, merely following the traditional edict of allowing the client to decide when he wishes to be bathed.

Respect the client's need for territoriality. Ask him for permission before looking in the bedside table for a basin. There is no need to store nursing care supplies in the one place in the client's room where he can keep his personal things. Ask him how he wears his hair and how he prefers to be addressed.

The nurse can discuss the plan of activities for the day with the client, pointing out his options and choices, and allow him to make decisions. Of course, the client's choices are limited by his disease and treatment regimen, but we can add to his sense of control of personal territory by asking permission when we must impose on that territory.

Encourage realistic optimism about his progress, with frequent orientations and references to the future. Plan, with the client and family, his convalescence and eventual return to productive life. Clarify any misconceptions so that the client comprehends his disease and its treatment. Establish continuity of care to minimize the impersonal and dehumanizing aspects of the environment. Emphasize the client's active role in his recovery, for instance, his role in coughing and deep breathing. If possible, spend time with the client, apart from nursing activities, to talk with him. Explain equipment and strange noises. Normalize the environment as much as possible. Control lighting, noise, and sights to minimize sensory overload.

Allow the client private time; whether he chooses to be alone or with significant others during that time is his decision. By familiarizing oneself with the client's psychodynamics and by being creative in one's nursing care, the critical care nurse can optimize the client's response to his illness.

NURSING CARE PLAN

Nursing Diagnosis: Alterations in protective mechanisms—Neutropenia
Medical Diagnosis: Neutropenia

Outcome. Signs and symptoms of infection will be minimized.

Nursing Interventions	Evaluation

1. Assess client every 4 hr for:
  a. temperature increase
  b. mouth: lesions, color changes, soreness, swelling
  c. rectum: tenderness, redness, induration, hemorrhoids
  d. GI: constipation, diarrhea, daily bowel check
  e. Skin: redness, swelling, induration, lesions, pain
  f. GU: pain, burning, odor
  g. respiratory: pain, cough, adventitious sounds, SOB
  h. Hickman site/central line: redness, swelling, tenderness, pain
	Client will display no signs or symptoms of infection.

2. Control environmental factors that could precipitate infection.
  a. strict handwashing
  b. no flowers, fresh fruit or vegetables
  c. screen visitors, staff for colds, fever, nausea, vomiting, varicella
  d. private room with door closed
  e. masks for people with upper respiratory infections	

Nursing Interventions   **Evaluation**

   f. masks for client and nurse when central line is entered

   g. no vases, or other standing collections of water

   h. strict aseptic technique in dressing changes, suctioning, pressure monitor lines, and central line tubing changes

   i. monitor housekeeping services given to client's room—damp dust with disinfectant, daily washing of floors and countertops with disinfectant

3. Prophylactic measures against infection—protect client's intact immune defenses.

   a. turn and position every hour

   b. keep skin clean and well lubricated by daily bath with mild soap and warm water, apply lotion every 3–4 hr

   c. monitor skin turgor every shift to assess hydration status of skin

   d. humidifier in room

   e. range of motion every 4 hr if client immobile

   f. change linens whenever soiled or wet

   g. pulmonary toilette (coughing, deep breathing, percussion, vibration, drainage, encentive spirometer) every 4 hr

4. Avoid invasive procedures—no injections, enemas, rectal temperatures.

5. Instruct client to avoid trauma.

   a. use electric razor

   b. avoid straining at stool

   c. report any signs or symptoms of infection

Nursing Diagnosis: Potential alterations in oral mucous membranes
Medical Diagnosis: Chemotherapy—Watch for stomatitis

Outcome. Client will have minimal or no oral mucous membrane problems.

Nursing Interventions	Evaluation
1. Assess daily for signs and symptoms mucositis: edema, pallor, erythema, increased temperature sensitivity, pain, ropy thick saliva, burning, ulcerations, lesions, candidiases.	Mucous membranes pink, intact, and painless.

Outcome. Client recognizes and reports signs and symptoms of mucositis and states appropriate preventative measures.

2. Institute preventative measures.
   a. instruct client to brush teeth twice daily with soft toothbrush or toothette
   b. use mild, nonabrasive toothpaste, floss twice daily when platelets $\geq$ 40^{000}/mm^3 and wbc $\geq$ 1500/mm^3
   c. rinse mouth with saline or saline and hydrogen peroxide (1:2 solution) 4 times a day
   d. avoid commercial mouth washes, hot spicy foods

Nursing Diagnosis: Alterations in Nutrition: Less than Body Requirements
Medical Diagnosis: Underweight

Outcome. Client will receive optimal protein and calories for height and weight.

Nursing Interventions	Evaluation
1. Obtain diet history, food preferences, weight, calorie count.	Client's weight will be appropriate for height and increased metabolic needs.
2. Encourage frequent, small feedings.	
3. Ensure client has mouth care prior to eating. Use viscous xylocaine prior to meal if client has stomatitis.	
4. Consult with dietitian weekly to ensure client is consuming optimal protein and calories.	

Nursing Diagnosis: Potential for ineffective coping
Medical Diagnosis:

Outcome: Client will: a) verbalize feelings related to his emotional state; b) identify his coping patterns and the consequences of the behavior that results; c) identify personal strengths and receive support through the nursing relationship; and d) make decisions and follow through with appropriate actions to change provocative situations in personal environment.

Nursing Interventions	Evaluation

1. Assess factors leading to potential for ineffective coping.

   a. environment
   b. illness
   c. change in role, self-concept, body image, sense of loss, forced dependency
   d. inadequate support system

2. Assess client's present coping status.

   a. determine onset of feelings and symptoms and their correlation with events and life changes
   b. assess ability to relate facts
   c. listen as client speaks to collect facts and observe facial expressions, gestures, eye contact, body positioning, tone, and intensity of voice
   d. demonstrate to client that you believe him and desire to help
   e. offer support as client talks
      i. reassure him that feelings he has must be difficult
      ii. when client is pessimistic, attempt to provide a more hopeful, realistic perspective

3. Teach constructive problem-solving techniques.

   a. assist person to problem solve in a constructive manner
      What is the problem?
      What are his options?
      What are advantages and disadvantages of each option?
   b. discuss possible alternatives— talk over problem with those involved
   c. assist client to identify problems that he cannot control directly and help him to practice stress-reducing activities for control (exercise, meditation)

4. Assist client to develop appropriate strategies based upon his personal

Evaluation (top right): Client will talk openly with nurse about feelings.

Nursing Interventions   Evaluation

strengths and previous experiences.
a. have client describe previous ex-
    periences with hospitalization
    and how he coped
b. encourage client to evaluate
    own behavior
c. be supportive of functional cop-
    ing behaviors
d. mobilize client to engage in
    activities he likes, e.g., arts and
    crafts
e. find outlets that foster feelings
    of personal achievement and
    self-esteem
    make time for relaxing activities
    stress relaxation activities

5. Correct lack of support systems.
    a. establish network of people who
        understand client
    b. decide who is best able to act as
        a support system with client
    c. maintain sense of humor with
        client
    d. allow tears

CHAPTER 9

Alterations in Protective Mechanisms: Increased Immune System Functions

The same immunological mechanisms that protect the individual can, conversely, damage normal tissue if the immune response is excessive or prolonged. Damage to normal cells and tissues occurs in autoimmune disease, for example, because immune responses are directed against parts of the client's body.

When the immune response and its corresponding inflammatory processes is exaggerated beyond its protective effects or is inappropriately directed toward a harmless material, the person is said to be hypersensitive. Allergy is defined as an altered state of immune reactivity and is a disorder of the immune system. Hypersensitivity and allergy are now used interchangeably.

Symptoms and signs of hyperimmune states are recognized by the presence of allergies and other immunological injury. Hypersensitivity reactions have been classified into four categories based on the nature of the antibody, the nature of the antigen, and indirectly the time course of the reaction (Table 9–1). Clinical manifestations of disease may be the consequence of one or any combination of these mechanisms of tissue injury.

TYPE I HYPERSENSITIVITY—ANAPHYLACTIC REACTIONS

Pathophysiology. Type I or anaphylactic reactions occur explosively within 5 to 15 minutes after antigen exposure. They are also known as immediate hypersensitivity reactions. They are B lymphocyte mediated and are characterized by the release of vasoactive substances from mast cells or basophils. Mast cells are found surrounding small veins in many areas of the body that are most frequently exposed to environmental antigens. Known as basophils when circulating in the blood, mast cells contain histamine, serotonin, slow-reacting substance of anaphylaxis (SRS-A), and other vasoactive substances capable of producing what is known as an anaphylactic type reaction in response to an antigen. The release of these active substances is due to the binding of the antigen to IgE antibodies, attached to mast cell and basophil surfaces.

TABLE 9-1. HYPERSENSITIVITY REACTIONS

	Type I Anaphylactic	Type II Cytotoxic	Type III Toxic Complex	Type IV Cell-mediated
Etiology and mechanism	Reagin (atopy) with antigen causes release of pharmacologic mediators of anaphylaxis from mast cells	Antibody combining with tissue antigens causes activation of complement system, which causes cytolysis	Antibody and soluble antigen form insoluble complexes that deposit at various sites causing inflammation, and cause activation of complement system	Immune lymphoid cell reaction with antigen K cells or proteins causes direct killing of antigenic cells, production of mediators of cell-mediated immune response causing accumulation of polymorphonuclear cells, monocytes, etc., The liberation of lysosomal enzymes and inflammation
Examples	Penicillin allergy, insect sting	Systemic lupus erythematosus, rheumatic fever	Serum sickness, chronic glomerulonephritis	Allograft rejection, poison ivy. Breakdown may lead to chronic mucocutaneous candidiasis, failure, or immune surveillance, and neoplasia

IgE is the antibody that is responsible for hypersensitivity. IgE circulates in body fluids, is attached to epithelial cells, and is also found fixed to mast cells in the body. The surface of a mast cell is packed with between 100,000 and 500,000 IgE receptors.

A clone of B lymphocytes is formed in response to an allergen, an antigen that would not ordinarily evoke an immune response but one to which the allergic client is about to become sensitive. Plasma cells from that clone produce antibodies against that allergen. These antibodies are of the IgE type. These IgE antibodies are, by necessity, specific to the allergen. A person is allergic to cats, for instance, because he makes IgE in response to the binding of a particular protein of cat hair or skin.

When specific IgE antibodies are synthesized by the millions in response to an allergen, they attach themselves to the mast cells. There is no allergic reaction yet. That happens when the individual next encounters that antigen. The antigen heads straight to the IgE fixed to mast cells and binds to the antibody. As a result the mast cell degranulates. Histamine, SRS-A, and eosinophil chemotactic factor of anaphylaxis are the major substances released from the mast cells during degranulation.

In addition to the mediators stored in the mast cells, there are two important groups of potent substances that are synthesized in most cells and also in leukocytes. These are the prostaglandins and the leukotrienes. The prostaglandins and the leukotrienes share a common origin. They are formed from arachidonic acid, which is a substance derived from cells, primarily white blood cells, whose membrane has been disrupted. The prostaglandins are a family of fatty acids whose importance as cellular messengers and as agents that affect various physiological processes have been known for quite a while. Some types of prostaglandins are potent but short-lived constrictors of smooth muscles in bronchi. Others, notably prostaglandin E_2, dilate bronchi. Other members of the prostaglandin family also affect the activity of mucous glands and the viscidity of their secretion, the stickiness of blood platelets, and the nonstick properties of the lining of blood vessels.

The leukotrienes have only recently been characterized chemically but their role in allergy was found many years ago. In the late 1930s, a substance was found in the extracellular fluid of the lung that was named the slow-reacting substance of anaphylaxis, or SRS-A. It causes a slow, long lasting and profound constriction of the airways in experimental animals, and is a mixture of three substances made of leukocytes. The leukotrienes are from 100 to 1000 times as potent as the prostaglandins or histamine in constricting the smallest airways of the bronchial tree. In allergy, the leukotrienes and the prostaglandins join with the mast cell mediators to give rise: to the contraction of smooth muscle in airways or intestine; to the dilation of small blood vessels, and an increase in their permeability to water and plasma proteins; to the secretion of thick, sticky mucous; and in the skin, to the stimulation of nerve endings that result in itching and pain.

Clinical Presentations and Nursing Assessments. Some individuals seem to possess certain HLA combinations that predispose to the hyperimmune sensitivity and result in an overt expression of the anaphylactic type reaction. There are two types of anaphylaxis. The type demonstrated clinically depends on the individual's genetic background, route of antigen access, and the target organ. Systemic anaphylaxis usually occurs with a large dose of antigen, given rapidly intravenously, intramuscularly, or subcutaneously. It is a generalized reaction with smooth muscle contraction, increased vascular permeability, hypotension, coagulopathies, specifically incoagulability of blood, decreased heart rate and complement levels. Some hypersensitive individuals develop circulatory shock and respiratory failure within minutes after injection of the specific antigen.

Cutaneous anaphylaxis is a localized reaction due to skin fixing of IgE. It is manifested in the skin and mucous membranes. Lesions occur in the skin, gastrointestinal tract, or nasal mucosa, and reach a maximum within 15 to 20 minutes after exposure to the antigen.

Medical Interventions. Early recognition and prompt treatment of anaphylaxis is imperative. Epinephrine is administered subcutaneously and intravenously in repeated doses until symptoms are abated. Volume expanders and vasopressive agents may be indicated in the presence of shock and hypotension, and oxygen therapy/ventilatory assistance may be indicated with respiratory insufficiency. Antihistamines and bronchodilators are given for urticaria–angioedema and bronchospasm, respectively. Corticosteroids are not effective for the acute event.

Nursing Interventions. Prevention is important. The client should attempt to avoid precipitating events, and may be desensitized. Desensitization is the process of injecting small amounts of antigen and gradually increasing the amount over a period of time.

Teaching and learning processes should be used in helping the client, because the environment and the emotional state of the individual will influence the severity of symptoms and effectiveness of treatment. Teaching the client environmental control and stress modulation are primary nursing activities.

TYPE II HYPERSENSITIVITY—CYTOTOXIC REACTIONS

Pathophysiology and Clinical Presentations. This type of hypersensitivity occurs as the result of antibodies, IgG or IgM, that react with antigens in tissues. The antigens may be intrinsic or result from binding of free antigens to the tissues. The tissue damage results from antigen–antibody reactions of the IgM type that activate the complement system. IgE antibodies can lead to tissue damage without activating the complement system. If a cell is the antigen and IgG the antibody, removal of the cell occurs by phagocytosis, usually by macrophages, and a deficiency of the cell type occurs. In other words, if the body does not recognize itself, it will develop antibodies and destroy native tissue. Cytotoxic reactions most commonly occur in the vascular system. If the target cells for this type of hypersensitivity is red blood cells, for instance, anemia will develop. The body perceives the red blood cells as an antigen, instead of recognizing it as self. A deficiency of red blood cells results as antibodies destroy them as antigens. If white blood cells are perceived as foreign, leukopenia develops; platelet destruction leads to thrombocytopenia. If endothelium is seen as foreign, a vascular purpura results. Cytotoxic reactions may involve any cell type in a particular tissue.

Examples of type II reactions include immune hemolytic anemia, transfusion reactions, systemic lupus erythematosus, erythroblastosis fetalis, and Goodpasture's syndrome.

The kidneys, particularly the glomerular basement membrane, because of its blood-filtering function, are quite vulnerable to this type of hypersensitivity. Goodpasture's syndrome and many other autoimmune diseases, for instance scleroderma, systemic lupus erythematosus, and polyarteritis nodosa all exhibit some cytotoxic phenomena of the kidneys.

Medical Interventions. Large volume plasmapheresis has been used recently in conjunction with immunosuppression to treat this type of hypersensitivity. The goal of plasmapheresis is to clear the blood of the excess antibodies that are causing the tissue damage. The body may perceive a sudden drop in antibody levels as problematic and could compensate by producing antibodies at a more rapid rate. The goal of concurrent immunosuppression is to prevent this phenomenon. The overall process tends to decrease the circulating levels of antibody and prevent further tissue damage.

Nursing Interventions. Nursing care for a client with this type of hypersensitivity is aimed at assisting him to cope with a chronic disease. The client needs to be informed about the nature of his disease. Despite the fact that his immune system is overproducing antibodies, he has a functional immunosuppression. Antibodies produced are consumed in attacking native tissue. The client should be aware that he is prone to infection, and institute preventative measures (see Chap. 8). In addition, medication teaching is vital in assisting the client to live with his illness. Early recognition of drug toxicities or disease complications hinge on the client's active participation on his health care, which is achieved through comprehensive understanding of disease and treatment. Emotional support should be provided to assist the client in coping with lifestyle changes and changes in self-esteem (see Chap. 8). Other nursing care measures are specific to the disease. For instance clients with systemic lupus erythematosus should understand that they cannot be in the sun without adequate protection without exacerbating their disease.

TYPE III HYPERSENSITIVITY—IMMUNE COMPLEX MEDIATED HYPERSENSITIVITY REACTIONS

Pathophysiology. The deposit of circulating antigen–antibody complexes in tissue leads to inflammation. Injury in immune complex disease is secondary to deposits of antigen–antibody complexes that create insoluble complexes around small blood vessels. The diseases thought to be immune complex diseases include systemic lupus erythematosus, bacterial endocarditis, and some malignancies. Immune complex disease may develop at a specific tissue site, such as connective tissue in rheumatoid arthritis or in the lung, as in hypersensitivity pneumonitis. The systemic form, like systemic lupus erythematosus, is characterized by immune complex deposits in various sites, such as the pleura, pericardium, blood vessels, and kidney.

The pathogenesis of this type of hypersensitivity lies in the complement system. The antigen–antibody complexes activate the complement system, which dilate blood vessels and attract neutrophils. The interaction of phagocytes and antigen–antibody complexes leads to the release of lysosomal enzymes with subsequent tissue damage. The complex is trapped in various areas of the body and elicits tissue damage. There is usually no tissue specificity for the immune complex. Ordinarily the reticuloendothelial system (RES) clears the immune complexes from the body. When it does not, immune complex disease results. This failure of the RES may be due to excessive amounts of immune complexes or defects in phagocytosis.

Clinical Presentations. There are two types of immune complex disease, the arthrus reaction and serum sickness. The arthrus reaction is extravascular. Antigen–antibody complexes are found in the skin and lead to edema, erythema, and hemorrhage within hours. The arthrus reaction is characterized by time, 2 to 5 hours, accumulation of neutrophils in the area, and an increase in vascular permeability. There is a localized ischemic thrombosis. Polyarteritis nodosa is a disorder with typical arthrus reactions distributed in vessels throughout the body. The arthrus reaction usually occurs when there is an excess of antibody.

The intravascular form of type III hypersensitivity is serum sickness. Here, immune complexes are formed in the blood, leading to vasculitis, arthritis, and glomerulonephritis. It has the same mechanism of action as the arthrus reaction. It most frequently occurs as a result of drug reactions or when transplant recipients receive antilymphocyte serum. It is usually associated with an excess of antigen. It may be caused by antibody production to an antigen, endogenously or exogenously, passive transfer of antibody or antigen, or the injection of preformed antigen–antibody complexes.

Both types of this reaction form toxic complexes that lead to necrotic tissue injury. Treatment and nursing care are similar to that for type II reaction.

TYPE IV HYPERSENSITIVITY—DELAYED TYPE REACTIONS

Pathophysiology and Clinical Presentations

HYPERSENSITIVITY. This is the only type of hypersensitivity reaction that is mediated by the cellular immune system. The other types of hypersensitivity are humorally mediated. It centers on the role of the killer T cell. Killer T cells are capable of killing bacteria, tumor cells, or other target cells after appropriate sensitization. They also release lymphokines, which stimulate phagocytes and other lymphocytes. Macrophages, attracted to the site, also cause tissue damage.

The most common example of delayed hypersensitivity reactions is the tuberculin skin test. Intradermal injection of old tuberculin will lead to erythema, induration, and other signs of inflammation in 24 to 48 hours in persons previously sensitized to the antigen.

Under normal circumstances, the T cells are able to evaluate the threat posed by an antigen and to distinguish between harmful substances and harmless ones. If this recognition system fails, a harmless substance may be mistaken for a harmful one. This harmless substance then acts as an antigen, provoking a cellular immune response. For example, when a person develops a contact dermatitis, a rash or other inflammation of the skin, after contact with a harmless material such as a necklace, the body has recognized this harmless substance as harmful. Treatment and nursing care is aimed at teaching the client to avoid the substances.

CHAPTER 10
Alterations in Protective Mechanisms: Disorders of Leukocytes

Leukocytes, or white blood cells, are the main constituent of the immune system. Therefore, disorders of this cell group lead to mortality and morbidity primarily from infection. Disorders of leukocytes can be broken down into three categories: leukemias, leukocytosis, and granulocytopenia.

LEUKEMIA

The leukemias are a group of neoplastic disorders involving cells of blood forming organs. There is a malignant transformation of the hematopoietic cells or their stem cells, with subsequent neoplastic proliferation of abnormal cells that are immature and hypofunctional. The proliferating abnormality is due to a new group of leukocytes; the basic defect seems to be the lack of normal maturation of the leukocytes. The leukemias are usually associated with abnormal leukocytes in the peripheral blood with replacement of normal bone marrow, leading to anemia, thrombocytopenia, and leukopenia. The incidence of leukemia is greater in adults, but progress in the treatment of leukemia has been greater in children.

The classification of leukemias is controversial. There are two schema of classification currently in use. The major leukemias are grouped into four basic types: acute myelocytic leukemia (AML); acute lymphocytic leukemia (ALL); chronic myelocytic leukemia (CML); and chronic lymphocytic leukemia (CLL). Acute leukemia is characterized by the undifferentiated morphology of the affected cell, which may be as undifferentiated as a blast cell. Acute leukemias are usually abrupt in onset and have a rapid disease progression. Chronic leukemia has a relative maturity of the affected cell, a gradual onset, and a prolonged clinical course. Subtypes within the classifications leads to other categories. In AML, for instance, the subtypes are: acute myeloblastic leukemia; acute myelomonocytic leukemia, acute promyelocytic leukemia,

TABLE 10-1. LEUKEMIA: FRENCH-AMERICAN-BRITISH (FAB) CLASSIFICATION

Acute Lymphoblastic Leukemia	
L1	Lymphoblastic leukemia
	Predominance of small lymphoblasts
	Childhood type
L2	Lymphoblastic leukemia
	Predominance of large lymphoblasts
	Heterogenous type
L3	Predominance of large, more primitive lymphoblasts
	Lymphoma type
Acute Non-Lymphoblastic Leukemia	
M0	Acute undifferentiated leukemia—AUL
	Not classifiable
M1	Acute myeloblastic leukemia—AML
	Without maturation—most common
	Less than 3% promyelocytes
M2	Acute myeloblastic leukemia—AML
	Some maturation
	More than 3% promyelocytes
M3	Acute promyelocytic leukemia—APL
	More than 30% promyelocytes
M4	Acute myelomonocytic leukemia—AMML
	Minor component-myelocyte or monocyte—is more than 20% in peripheral blood and/or BM
M5a	Acute monocytic leukemia—AMOL
	Poorly differentiated
M5b	Acute monocytic leukemia—AMOL
	Differentiated
M6	Erythroleukemia

acute monocytic leukemia, and erythroleukemia, all based on cellular differentiation (Table 10–1).

The leukemias found in the adult are AML, ALL, CML, and CLL. AML usually affects people from the third decade to old age. ALL, in the adult, is more frequent after age 65. CML and CLL are also more common in the older adult. Sixty percent of all leukemias are acute (Table 10–2).

There are many theories about the cause of leukemia. It may be an immunological defect, viral infection, or have a genetic basis. The hypothesis most widely accepted is that a clone of leukemic cells probably develops from

TABLE 10-2. INCIDENCE OF LEUKEMIA

AML—	Third decade to old age
ALL—	Children and after age 65
CML—	Older adult
CLL—	Older adult

a single cell mutation. The clone has a longer generation time than normal marrow cells, but produces few, if any, endstage cells. Leukemic cells retain their ability to divide, but fail to mature and differentiate. Leukemic cells have a prolonged total life and a prolonged reproductive life so they remain immature for a longer period of time than normal cells. Consequently, despite a slow doubling time, leukemic cells infiltrate bone marrow, lymph nodes, spleen, and other organs and tissues. The most commonly considered causal factors include: congenital conditions especially Down's syndrome, which is associated with increased incidences of ALL and AML; exposure to certain chemicals; and exposure to large doses of radiation.

Clinical Presentations and Nursing Assessments. ALL is most common in childhood, and represents less than 10 percent of adult leukemias. Meningeal leukemia is frequently associated with ALL, producing headache, nausea, vomiting, paresis, enuresis, visual disturbances, papilledema, cranial nerve palsies, seizures, and coma. Leukostatic thrombi associated with circulating blast cells of more than 100,000 lead to intracerebral hemorrhage. Intracerebral bleeding is found in association with severe thrombocytopenia. Remission is achieved with multidrug therapy in 65 to 80 percent of adults. The majority relapse within 3 years.

AML is the most common type of leukemia in young adults. It responds much less favorably to therapy than ALL. 70 percent achieve a remission, which lasts anywhere from 6 months to 2 years. There are two reasons why AML is less responsive to chemotherapy than other leukemias. There is no cytotoxic drug that kills the leukemic myeloblasts without also being toxic to the normal hematopoietic precursors. Because those precursors are already diminished by disease, the drug therapy is doubly harmful to the client. Also, there are fewer drugs or drug combinations in use that are able to kill the leukemic cells rather than the lymphoblasts.

Coagulation abnormalities are common in AML. This is especially true in one subtype of AML, acute promyelocytic leukemia (APML). There is a frequent association of severe hemorrhagic diatheses caused by thrombocytopenia and disseminated intravascular coagulation (DIC) with APML. This is due to a release of procoagulant materials by leukocytic granules, depletion of various coagulation factors, and abnormal amounts of fibrin split products (FSP) in the blood. Some institutions are offering a bone marrow transplantation to appropriate clients with AML. The transplant is done during the first remission. The rationale for doing a bone marrow transplant is that the long-term remission rate is so low.

The chronic leukemias are more regulated processes, and are quite responsive to chemotherapy. After a variable period of 2 to 5 years in remission, more than 70 percent of patients with CML develop an acute phase known as a blastic crisis. This is a particularly resistant form of acute leukemia, and with few exceptions, death results. Both types of chronic leukemia are most frequently encountered in the older adult.

TABLE 10-3. CHARACTERISTICS OF LEUKEMIA

ALL—	Depressed hematopoiesis Blasts in bone marrow
AML—	Depressed hematopoiesis Blasts in bone marrow Auer bodies
CML—	Splenomegaly, ↑WBC ↓Leukocyte acid, phosphatase Philadelphia chromosome
CLL—	Hypogammaglobulinemia Lymphadenopathy

Laboratory Studies. Diagnosis of AML and ALL is made by noting presenting symptoms of depressed hematopoiesis: bleeding tendency, ecchymoses, petechiae, frequent infections, pallor, and fatigue. Peripheral blood reveals decreased hemoglobin and platelet counts. White blood cell counts may be low, normal, or elevated. The bone marrow is dominated by leukemic blasts of the affected cell line. The presence of Auer bodies is diagnostic of AML, as is the Philadelphia chromosome of CML. In CML, there is abnormal proliferation of relatively mature granulocytes that accumulate in the blood, bone marrow, and organs. Splenomegaly, increased leukocytes with an increase in eosinophils and basophils, and a low leukocyte acid phosphatase are signs of CML. In CLL, the neoplastic cell resembles a normal B lymphocyte but does not respond to antigen stimulation. As a result, the individual has hypogammaglobulinemia and lymphadenopathy (Table 10-3).

Medical Interventions. Treatment of the leukemias is with multidrug regimens of chemotherapy (see Chap. 7). Modern multidrug chemotherapy, used to induce remissions in leukemia, almost universally produces a phase of bone marrow destruction or hypocellularity. Theoretically, then, the bone marrow repopulates with normal cells. It is during the phase of marrow cellularity secondary to chemotherapy that most of the problems will be seen in the acute setting. These problems are: nursing care of the immunosuppressed client; nursing care of the client with bleeding disorders; psychosocial adaptation of the client who is immunosuppressed; and nutrition as discussed in other sections of this text.

Sepsis is a frequent finding in clients with leukemia, and carries a high mortality rate. If infection does develop, it must be recognized early and treated aggressively.

Hyperuricemia is a complication of many chemotherapeutic regimens in leukemic clients. It is more often pronounced during the rapid lysis of leukemic cells that accompanies intensive chemotherapy. The precipitation of uric acid crystals in the kidney structures can lead to renal failure, manifested by lethargy, nausea and vomiting, hematuria, renal pain, oliguria, or anuria.

Allopurinol is given prophylactically to decrease the production of uric acid. Sodium bicarbonate is also used to alkalinize the urine, preventing the formation of acid crystals. The client must be well hydrated to reduce the concentration of uric acid in the urine.

Nursing Interventions. A diagnosis of leukemia is a threat to the client's sense of self. He is confronted with the reality of death, and a vigorous therapeutic regimen, with all of its associated changes in body image, independence, and alterations in life-style. The nurse caring for this client and his family must help them redefine priorities, understand the illness and its treatment, and to find hope.

LEUKOCYTOSIS

Leukocytosis is a leukocyte count of more than 10,000 per cu mm with an increase in circulating neutrophils, bands, and occasionally metamyelocytes. It is a common finding and can be relative or absolute. Leukocytosis is caused by five primary situations (Table 10–4):

1. Bacterial infections, especially with pyogenic bacteria.
2. Inflammation or tissue necrosis, for instance infarction, myositis, vasculitis.
3. Intoxications, for instance uremia, eclampsia, acidosis, gout.
4. Neoplasms, especially bronchogenic carcinoma, lymphoma, melanoma.
5. Other conditions, for instance acute hemorrhage or hemolysis, especially in children, postsplenectomy.

Granulocytes are produced on demand and the body can pour them out in the presence of infection or stress. A demand for granulocytes imposed by peripheral bacterial invasion is met at first by the egress into the tissues of cells from the marginal circulating pool of granulocytes. Release of bone marrow reserves is then accelerated. Finally there is an increased rate of cell proliferation in the marrow. Abnormal features associated with leukocytosis include a shift to the left in blood leukocytes. A shift to the left is a rise in the ratio of nonsegmented to segmented neutrophils, or immature neutrophils, due to

TABLE 10-4. CAUSES OF LEUKOCYTOSIS

1. Bacterial infections, especially with pyogenic bacteria
2. Inflammation or tissue necrosis—infarction, myositis, vasculitis
3. Metabolic intoxications—uremia, eclampsia
4. Neoplasms
5. Other—acute hemorrhage, hemolysis, post-splenectomy

the increased rate of cell production in the marrow. Fever is seen in leuko-cytosis from leukocyte pyrogen. Treatment for leukocytosis is to treat the under-lying disease.

GRANULOCYTOPENIA

Granulocytopenia indicates decreased numbers of circulating granulocytes. Agranulocytosis describes a more severe form, less than 300 granulocytes/μl. Leukopenia means depression of the total leukocyte count. Neutropenia is a near synonym for granulocytopenia. The risk of infection is significantly in-creased when granulocytes are less than 1000/μl. Granulocytopenia may be due to decreased production, to increased destruction, congenital defects, or viral infections.

Decreased Production of Granulocytes

Granulocytopenia, because of a diminished production of granulocytes, arises from an inadequate level of granulopoiesis to maintain a normal level of gran-ulocytes. Major underlying causes are: aplastic anemia; myelophthisis from invading cancer cells, fibrosis, and granulomas; cytotoxic chemotherapeutic agents that, by intention or nonintention, depress the production of granulo-poietic cells; and ineffective granulopoiesis such as occurs in megaloblastic anemia.

Granulocytopenia in these instances results in decreased availability of cells. Marrow storage and marginal granulocyte pools are decreased and the mobilization of neutrophils at the inflammatory site is impaired. Neutrophil survival is normal.

Increased Destruction of Granulocytes

Granulocytopenia in this category is due to abnormal cell destruction or in-creased cell utilization. Major causes are: early infection before the new cells from the marrow are produced; leukapheresis; hypersplenism; leukoagglutinins secondary to the administration of certain drugs; or leukocyte antibodies, es-pecially following multiple blood transfusions and systemic lupus erythematosus. Hypersplenism can cause increased destruction of granulocytes. Splenic sequestration of granulocytes due to splenomegaly or almost any cause may lead to granulocytopenia. Infiltration of the spleen with lymphoma or leukemia, and congestive splenomegaly secondary to portal cirrhosis all can provide the anatomical basis for increased granulocytic sequestration. Leuko-agglutinins secondary to drugs such as aminopyrine and propylthiouracil can lead to increased destruction of granulocytes as well. The destruction of ag-glutinated granulocytes occurs in the lung as well as in other sites. Granulocyte precursors also may be affected. Bone marrow examination will show decreased myelocytes and myeloblasts. The drug forms a complex with the leukocyte and becomes antigenic. Antibody is elicited which is active only against the complex. In the absence of the drug, the antibody remains in the plasma in an inactive form. Subsequent administration of drug to a sensitized individual activates antibody on the neutrophil surface. The result is massive leukoagglutination with pulmonary sequestration and removal of granulocytes from the circulation. Compensatory myeloid hyperplasia then occurs in the marrow. Continued drug administration leads to marrow exhaustion.

Congenital Defects of Granulocytes

Congenital defects include chronic granulomatous disease, Chédiak–Higashi syndrome, May–Hegglin anomaly, and Alder–Reilly bodies. Chronic granulomatous disease is an inherited disorder seen in children. The children will have recurrent infections with organisms of low pathogenicity, suppurative granulomas with pneumonia, suppurating lymph nodes, and hepatosplenomegaly. Chédiak–Higashi syndrome is also a hereditary disorder characterized by abnormal lysosomes in many cell types. Defective granulocytes contain large inclusion bodies that are defective primary granules. The client has a defective pigment metabolism, characterized by oculocutaneous albinism, neurological abnormalities, and a high incidence of lymphoreticular neoplasms. Affected children have recurrent infections due to a variety of bacteria. The May–Hegglin anomaly is an inherited disorder associated with thrombocytopenia, giant platelets, and a variably severe bleeding tendency. Inclusion bodies are present in the granulocytes. Alder–Reilly bodies are large granulations found in the Alder–Reilly anomaly, a recessively inherited disorder, or in patients with the Hurler syndrome, the Hunter syndrome, or other forms of dwarfism. These inclusions do not appear to interfere with granulocyte function.

Viral Infections

Granulocytopenia may occur during viral infections, and after severe acute bacterial infections with septicemia. This may be due to a combination of decreased production and increased destruction of granulocytes. The bone marrow production of granulocytes is overwhelmed by the infection while the existent cells are utilized in fighting off the infection.

Clinical Effects

The clinical syndromes associated with granulocytopenia are caused by inadequate bacterial phagocytosis and increased susceptibility to bacterial infection. Infections, acute and chronic, and mucous membrane ulceration are the common features. The most dramatic illustration of this tendency is seen in acute drug-induced agranulocytosis. At first, there are few symptoms, but within a day or two clients develop sore throat, fever, chills, necrosis of oral mucous membranes, and bacteremia. When severe neutropenia results from leukocyte destruction, fever is due to pyrogen. However, susceptibility to infection is common with neutropenia of any cause. Vulnerability to infection becomes serious when the neutrophil count falls below 1000 per cu mm and very serious when below 500 per cu mm. Nursing care is aimed at preventing infection (see Chap. 8).

CHAPTER 11

Alteration in Oxygenation: Disorders of Erythrocytes

There are numerous disorders that affect the red blood cells (RBC). Anemia is the most common condition resulting from hematopoietic disease.

ANEMIA

Anemia is usually defined as a reduction below the normal level in the number of RBCs, the quantity of hemoglobin, and the volume of packed RBCs per hundred milliliters of blood. Anemia is not a diagnostic entity but a clinical sign. Although it is not a specific disease, it is the principal manifestation of a number of abnormal conditions such as deficiency states caused by a dietary lack of iron, vitamin B_{12}, and folic acid, hereditary disorders of the erythrocyte, disorders involving the hematopoietic tissues (bone marrow damage or a hyperactive spleen), and bleeding from the gastrointestinal tract because of cancer or hemorrhage from any organ.

The incidence of anemia is extremely high. This is particularly true in underdeveloped countries where nutrition is poor. Some epidemiologists calculate that at least one half of the world's population suffers from anemia at some time.

The major role of erythrocytes is to transport oxygen to the tissue. Consequently, the major physiological effect of anemia is to reduce the capacity of the client's blood to carry oxygen to the tissue. This results in tissue hypoxia. Tissue hypoxia is the basic underlying cause of all symptoms accompanying anemia.

Tissue hypoxia, occurring when oxygen is not available or is insufficient at the cellular levels for metabolic activity, leads to many compensatory mechanisms. Many of the signs and symptoms of anemia are also related to the compensatory mechanisms called into action to prevent destructive tissue hypoxia.

Compensatory Mechanisms

On the cellular level, in anemia, there is an increased synthesis of 2,3-DPG that shifts the oxyhemoglobin dissociation curve to the right. In this way, more oxygen is released to the tissues at a higher oxygen tension. Compensation also occurs by the use of all potential capillary channels to increase tissue perfusion to vital areas, at the expense of nonvital donor areas. Major donor areas for redistribution of blood are the skin and the kidneys. Vasoconstriction occurs, with clinical findings of pallor. There is also a shift away from the kidneys. Although the kidneys are vital organs, under normal conditions, the oxygen supply to the kidneys is in excess of its demand. Even in severe anemia, with renal blood flow reduced by about 50 percent, reduction in renal function may be only mildly or moderately curtailed.

A high cardiac output is another excellent compensatory mechanism that increases tissue oxygenation, but it may also increase metabolic needs. Cardiac output does not measurably increase in chronic anemia until hemoglobin level reach 7 g. Signs of compensatory cardiac activity include tachycardia, systolic flow murmur, and orthostatic hypotension. The normal heart will sustain hyperactivity for prolonged periods. However, angina and high output heart failure may occur if coronary oxygen demands are not filled, or if there is preexisting coronary disease. It is important to note that in chronic anemia, the blood volume is normal because of increased plasma volume. An increased respiratory rate occurs also in an attempt to increase oxygenation. This accounts for symptoms of exertional dyspnea and orthopnea.

There is an increase in the rate of RBC production as determined by an increase in reticulocyte count. There is also increased production of erythropoietin as a physiological response to renal hypoxia. When the bone marrow is capable of responding, the client's clinical complaints may be generalized aches and pains or sternal tenderness.

When these compensatory mechanisms are unable to correct the tissue hypoxia, symptoms on this basis alone occur. The client may present with angina, intermittent claudication, and night cramps due to muscle tissue hypoxia. Also, he may have headaches, light-headedness, roaring in the ears, faintness, irritability and depression (Table 11–1).

TABLE 11-1. COMPENSATORY MECHANISMS IN ANEMIA

Compensation	Clinical Effects

↑ Synthesis of 2,3-DPG
   redistribution of blood
	More oxygen released to tissue
	   ↓ blood flow to kidneys, skin
	   → pallor, ↓ urine output

↑ Cardiac output	Tachycardia, systolic flow murmur, orthostatic hypotension
↑ Respiratory rate	Exertional dyspnea, orthopnea
↑ Production of erythropoietin	↑ RBC production, generalized aches and pains, sternal tenderness

TABLE 11-2. CLASSIFICATION OF ANEMIA

Decreased hemoglobin synthesis	Blood loss
Iron deficiency	Increased destruction of RBC
Thalassemia	Abnormal hemoglobins (sickle cell
Lead poisoning	anemia)
Sideroblastic anemia	Defective glycolysis (G6PD deficiency)
Nuclear-cytoplasmic defects	Membrane abnormalities (spherocytosis)
Vitamin B_{12} deficiency	Physical causes (prosthetic heart
Folate deficiency	valves)
Pernicious anemia	Immunological causes
Decreased RBC precursors	Infectious agents
Aplastic anemia	Hypersplenism
Myelofibrosis	Vasculitis
Marrow toxins	Osmotic injury
Decreased erthropoietin effect	
Anemia of chronic disease	

CLASSIFICATION OF ANEMIA

Anemia can be secondary to blood loss. It can also be the result of a decreased production of erythrocytes. Decreased hemoglobin synthesis, for instance iron deficiency, thalassemias, lead poisoning, and sideroblastic anemia, nuclear–cytoplasmic defects, as in vitamin B_{12} and folate deficiencies, decreased RBC precursors, as in aplastic anemia, myelofibrosis, and marrow toxins, decreased erythropoietin effect, as in anemias of chronic disease are all situations that decrease the production of erythrocytes (Table 11-2).

Anemia can result from an increased destruction of RBCs. This can be intrinsic to erythrocytes as in abnormal hemoglobins, defective glycolysis such as G6PD deficiency, and membrane abnormalities such as hereditary spherocytosis or elliptocytosis. Increased RBC destruction can also result from sources extrinsic to erythrocytes: physical causes such as prosthetic heart valves or thrombotic thrombocytopenia purpura; antibodies as in immune thrombocytopenic purpura; infectious agents and toxins; or other causes such as hypersplenism, vasculitis syndromes, or osmotic and physical injury.

DIAGNOSIS OF ANEMIA

A careful history should be obtained. Is the anemia of acute onset or congenital? Is there a history of excessive blood loss; evidence of melena, hematemesis, hematuria; familial incidence of anemia; alcohol or drug use; or underlying disease? Review exposure to medications and potentially harmful industrial or household toxins. Obtain a diet history for evidence of decreased intake of iron, folic acid, or vitamin B_{12}.

Laboratory studies to be obtained include hematocrit (Hct) and hemoglobin (Hgb), RBC morphology, and variations in Hgb content. Micro-

TABLE 11-3. DIAGNOSIS OF ANEMIA

System	Signs and Symptoms
CV/Respiratory	Exertional dyspnea, tachycardia, tachypnea, palpitations, cardiac enlargement, angina, murmurs, claudication, dependent edema, orthopnea, nocturia, bounding, arterial pulses, capillary pulsations, vascular bruits
Neuromuscular	Headache, faintness, vertigo, tinnitus, bone tenderness (sternum), loss of concentration, fatigue, cold sensitivity
Skin	Pallor (mucous membranes and nailbeds), pale palm lines, delayed wound healing, purpura, jaundice, pruritis, spider angiomas
GI	Anorexia, nausea, flatulence, constipation, diarrhea
GU	Menstrual irregularity, amenorrhea, menorrhagia, loss of libido or potency

cytic RBCs are smaller than normal; macrocytic are larger than normal. Microcytosis, especially with hypochromia, is suggestive of defective Hgb synthesis; macrocytosis strongly suggests megaloblastic anemia, vitamin B_{12} and folate deficiencies. A normally hemoglobinized RBC is normochromic; hypochromic RBC are poorly hemoglobinized. Mean corpuscular hemoglobin (MCH) and mean corpuscular hemoglobin concentration (MCHC) measure the hemoglobin concentration in RBCs. Hypochromic RBCs are usually microcytic and are seen in disorders of hemoglobin synthesis, for instance iron deficiency, thalassemia, and sideroblastic anemia (see Table 11-3 and Chap. 1).

Signs and symptoms of anemia affect every system of the body (Table 11-4).

- *Cardiovascular and respiratory:* exertional dyspnea, tachycardia, palpitations, angina, claudication, orthopnea, bounding arterial pulses, capillary pulsation, vascular bruits, cardiac englargement, murmurs, dependent edema, nocturia, and tachypnea.
- *Neuromuscular:* headache, vertigo, faintness, tinnitus, bone tenderness especially of the sternum, loss of concentration, fatigue, cold sensitivity.
- *Skin:* pallor, particularly the mucous membranes and nailbeds, pale palm lines, delayed wound healing, purpura, jaundice, pruritis, spider angiomas.
- *Genitourinary:* menstrual irregularity, amenorrhea, loss of libido or potency.

Decreased Hemoglobin Synthesis

Iron Deficiency Anemia
Iron deficiency anemia can be secondary to blood loss from the gastrointestinal, ureterovaginal, or respiratory tracts; to increased internal demands, for in-

TABLE 11-4. SIGNS AND SYMPTOMS CHARACTERIZED BY BLOOD DYSCRASIAS

Signs and Symptoms	Bases
Chronic fatigue and dyspnea	↓ In erythrocytes (anemias, leukemias, hemorrhagic disorders). Causes a reduction in the oxygen carrying capacity of the blood
Increased susceptibility to infection	↓ In mature circulating leukocytes (leukemia, leukopenia, lymphoma). Decreases number of cells available to combat invading microorganisms and produce antibodies
GI symptoms—anorexia, weight loss, indigestion, sore mouth and tongue	↓ In gastric secretions (as seen in pernicious anemia). Abnormal changes in mucous membrane cells and the effects of certain drugs and extreme fatigue all contribute to lack of desire or inability to eat
Hemorrhage and bleeding into tissue and joints, and from mucous membranes	Hemorrhage results either from a ↓ in platelet count (as result of drugs, infections, or autoimmune causes) or from absence of one or more clotting factors
Bone pain and deformity	Hyperactivity of bone marrow (seen in myeloproliferative disorders) and pathlogical fractures (seen in many cancers) both produce bone pain and deformity
Jaundice	Rupture and hemolysis of abnormal erythrocytes (characteristics of hemolytic anemias and pernicious anemia) cause release of large amounts of bilirubin into the circulation
Enlarged liver and spleen, and hyperplasia of bone marrow	Caused by either: congestion from over production of cells (polycythemia, leukemia, etc.), or excessive demands upon these organs to destroy defective cells (e.g., hemolytic anemias)
Mental depression	Chronic depression may result from the chronicity of most blood diseases and the fatigue and discomfort characteristic of these disorders

stance in pregnancy, infancy, adolescence, or in polycythemias; from malabsorption, as in celiac sprue, partial or total gastrectomy; or from dietary inadequacy. In this and related disorders, the basic defect appears to be a decreased supply to the developing RBC of a crucial component of hemoglobin, iron, essential to the oxygen carrying function of heme. When these disorders of heme synthesis become severe, the marrow produces RBCs that are deficient in hemoglobin concentration, hypochromic and microcytic.

Pathophysiology. The adult body contains about 50 mg of iron per 100 ml of blood. Total body iron ranges between 2 and 6 g, depending upon the size of the individual and the amount of Hgb the client's cells contain. Approximately two-thirds of this iron is contained in Hgb; the other third is stored in the bone marrow, spleen, liver, and muscle. If an individual develops an iron deficiency, the iron stores are depleted first, followed later by a reduction in Hgb formation.

We obtain iron from food; important sources are liver (the richest source), oysters, lean meat, kidney beans, whole wheat bread, kale, spinach, egg yolk, turnip tops, beet greens, carrots, apricots, and raisins.

An adequate diet supplies the body with about 12 to 15 mg of iron per day, of which only 5 to 10 percent is absorbed. The amount of iron normally absorbed daily is just sufficient to meet the needs of healthy men and older women past the childbearing age, but is not sufficient to supply the greater needs of menstruating and pregnant women, adolescents, infants, and children. These five groups must have a higher daily intake of iron if iron deficiency is to be prevented. Fortunately, if iron intake is inadequate during childhood or pregnancy or if bleeding develops, the gastrointestinal tract is capable of increasing the absorption of iron to around 20 to 30 percent of the total daily intake.

Iron is excreted in urine, sweat, bile, feces, and from the skin of desquamated cells. Daily iron excretion is normally less than 1 mg. The normal menses causes women to lose another 12 to 30 mg monthly. The only abnormal source of iron loss is hemorrhage or chronic bleeding. A chronic blood loss of 2 to 4 ml per day can result in iron deficiency anemia because 1 mg of iron is lost in every 2 ml of blood.

Clinical Presentations and Nursing Assessments. In mild cases, the client is asymptomatic. However, in more severe cases all the general symptoms of anemia discussed earlier appear. Later in the course of disease, clients usually develop brittleness of hair and nails. In severe cases, the client may experience dysphagia, stomatitis, and atrophic glossitis (tongue is inflamed and smooth due to atrophy or papillae).

Laboratory Studies. The diagnosis is made by a histochemical estimation of macrophage iron stores in aspirated bone marrow, which shows depleted body iron stores. Serum iron levels are decreased, and the platelet count is often increased. Serum iron binding capacity is increased. There is a newly available commercial test that involves an immunoradiametric assay of the serum for ferritin. In clients with iron deficiency anemia, levels are below normal. Once the diagnosis of iron deficiency anemia is made, studies are conducted to find the cause of the anemia.

Medical Interventions. Therapeutic goals for clients with iron deficiency anemia are to diagnose and correct the underlying cause of the anemia, and to correct the iron deficit by means of medicinal iron preparations and a diet high in food iron.

Medicinal iron can be administered orally or parenterally; however, it is administered orally whenever possible. The drugs of choice for oral administration are ferrous sulfate or ferrous gluconate.

It is important to administer oral iron preparations correctly. First, because iron salts are gastric irritants, they should always be given following meals or a snack. Second, undiluted liquid preparations of iron salts stain the teeth. Liquid iron should be well diluted and administered through a straw. Third, whenever possible, give ferrous salts with orange juice because ascorbic acid promotes better iron absorption. Finally, warn the clients that iron preparations change the color of stools because iron is excreted in bowel movements.

Parenteral iron therapy is given to clients who have an intolerance to oral iron preparations, who habitually forget to take their medications, or who are continuing to suffer from blood losses. Iron dextran is the drug of choice. Iron dextran causes darkening and discoloration of the skin around the injection site unless administered by Z-track injection technique. A favorable response to iron therapy typically occurs within 48 hours.

Nursing care is aimed at caring for an anemic client (see Chap. 13) and diet teaching.

Thalassemia

The thalassemias are a heterogeneous and complex group of inherited disorders of hemoglobin synthesis characterized by absent or diminished synthesis of one of the globin chains of Hgb A. Clinical manifestations depend upon whether the afflicted individual is homozygous or heterozygous for the thalassemia trait. Thalassemia major and intermedia, characterized by a profound anemia, appear in homozygotes. Thalassemia minor is characterized by a relatively mild anemia and develops in heterozygotes. The disease is most prevalent in Mediterranean populations and in Orientals, and is also known as Cooley's anemia.

Pathophysiology. Hemoglobin is composed of two pairs of polypeptide chains, alpha chains and beta chains. Either alpha or beta chains can be affected by diminished synthesis. The polypeptide chains are completely normal in structure, but an insufficient amount of polypeptide chains exist as a result of the genetic defect. In alpha thalassemia, alpha chain synthesis is slowed; in beta thalassemia, beta chain synthesis is retarded.

Beta thalassemia is by far the most common form of the disease and is simply referred to as "thalassemia." Some clients with this disorder have no Hgb A whatsoever, only Hgb S and the minor Hgbs.

Clinical Presentations and Nursing Assessments. The symptoms of thalassemia major are generally the same as those of other hemolytic anemias—jaundice, cholelithiasis, leg ulcers, and enlarged spleen. The disease can be detected early in infancy. Characteristic RBC changes often can be recognized by 6 weeks of age. Poor growth and development due to chronic anemia, and skeletal changes of the skull, long bones, and hands due to intense, ineffective marrow erythroid hyperplasia are common. The children are subject to recurrent infections, and develop hemosiderosis. This results primarily from iron deposition from transfused blood, but the anemia itself accelerates iron uptake and its deposition in parenchymal tissue. Siderosis in the myocardium causes conduction defects and heart failure. Heart disease is overwhelmingly the cause of death of affected clients in childhood or early life. Clinically the ineffective erythropoiesis leads to erythroid hyperplasia causing severe medullary expansion and remodeling of bone. This causes the skeletal lesions described and a striking chipmunk-like or mongoloid facial appearance due to marrow hyperplasia and expansion of facial bones. Extension extramedullary erythropoiesis produces massive hepatosplenomegaly, and accelerated bilirubin production predisposes the client to biliary tract disease.

Laboratory Studies. Laboratory findings in thalassemia include: target cells (abnormally thin fragile cells) and other bizarrely shaped erythrocytes; serum bilirubin and fecal and urinary urobilinogen are greatly elevated because of the severe hemolysis; Hgb F (fetal hemoglobin) is greatly elevated; Hgb A_2 (a normal variant of Hgb A) is also elevated. The client will have a hypochromic anemia with marked poikilocytosis (variability in RBC shape), ineffective erythropoiesis, and accelerated hemolysis.

The high percentages of Hgb F and Hgb A_2 are a result of the decrease in beta chains characteristic of this anemia, which forces the bone marrow to produce abnormally large numbers of alpha chains, gamma chains (which are normally made only during fetal life), and delta chains. The compensatory increase in Hgb F results from the combination of alpha and gamma chains, whereas the increase in Hgb A_2 results from the combination of alpha and delta chains.

Medical Interventions. The treatment of children with this disorder is difficult. Growth and mental retardation may be controlled by regular blood transfusions but this accelerates the development of life threatening hemosiderosis or iron overload. Continuous subcutaneous infusion of iron-chelating agents for prevention of siderosis recently has been shown to lead to negative overall iron balance in these clients. Splenectomy is considered when rapid splenic sequestration of transfused RBCs increase the rate of transfusion requirements.

Nursing Interventions. Care of the anemic client has been discussed elsewhere. For this particular client, attention should be directed at assisting the client and his family in coping with a chronic disease and life long transfusion therapy.

Other Thalassemias

Thalassemia minor is usually asymptomatic with the exception of a mild anemia.

Alpha thalassemias are the consequence of partial or complete suppression of normal alpha chain synthesis. When one alpha gene is affected, the client is said to manifest the silent carrier state, with no hematologic or clinical abnormalities. It is detected only by studies of reticulocyte globin chain synthesis. The most severe form of alpha thalassemia is called hydrops fetalis, with all four alpha genes inactive. The affected fetusus are hydropic from severe anemia and congestive heart failure, and are born dead or die shortly thereafter.

Prenatal diagnosis of many genetic disorders is now possible and offers an alternative to these potentially tragic disorders.

Nuclear Cytoplasmic Defects

Megaloblastic Anemias

The megaloblastic anemias are due to a defect in DNA synthesis, most commonly caused by lack of coenzymes required for DNA synthesis. The missing coenzyme is usually one of two vitamins, folic acid (folate) or vitamin B_{12} (cobalamin).

Pathophysiology. Vitamin B_{12}, which contains cobalt, has two major functions: it is essential for normal RBC maturation and it is necessary for normal nervous system function. Dietary sources of vitamin B_{12} are animal products such as liver, milk, and eggs. It is also produced by bacteria within the intestines of humans and animals. Other names for vitamin B_{12} are cyanocobalamin and extrinsic factor. The extrinsic factor (vitamin B_{12} obtained from foods) cannot be absorbed by the small intestine unless a substance known as the intrinsic factor is present.

Folic acid is also necessary for RBC formation and maturation. It does not play a role in nervous system function. The major dietary sources of folic acid are green vegetables and liver.

Anemias due to deficiencies of vitamin B_{12} and folic acid are called megaloblastic anemias because they are characterized by the appearance of megaloblasts (large primitive erythrocytes) in blood and bone marrow. Other common features are the development of leukopenia and thrombocytopenia; oral, gastrointestinal, and neurological symptoms; and a favorable response to injections of either vitamin B_{12} or folic acid.

The underlying defects in megaloblastic anemias are disturbed synthesis of DNA. Deficiencies of either vitamin B_{12} or folic acid eventually impede the formation of essential DNA precursors. As a result, maturation of erythrocytes, leukocytes, and platelets is defective.

When folic acid of vitamin B_{12} is lacking, other cells with high turnover rates, which must make DNA in order to replicate, also may be affected. Serum unconjugated bilirubin may be increased due to release of hemoglobin from RBC precursors destroyed in bone marrow. Therefore, these disorders are characterized by ineffective erythropoiesis. For unknown reasons, megaloblastic erythroid precursors contain large amounts of lactic dehydrogenase (LDH), therefore LDH levels are increased. Many megaloblasts die in the bone marrow. There is marked hyperplasia of erythroid precursor compartment of the bone marrow but few reticulocytes. Howell-Jolly bodies are common, which are small nuclear remnants seen after splenectomy, severe hemolytic anemias, and in ineffective erythropoiesis. Neutrophils are hypersegmented.

Clinical Presentations and Nursing Assessments. To differentiate vitamin B_{12} anemia from folate deficiency, one must look for neurological findings. In vitamin B_{12} deficiency, the client may have a loss of position and vibration sense in the extremities. Folate deficiency does not result in these neurological signs. One must also look at serum vitamin concentrations. Both vitamin B_{12} and folate levels are measured by radioisotopic methods.

Folate deficiency is caused by inadequate diet by parenteral alimentation, by poor diet associated with alcohol ingestion, small intestine disease for instance gluten sensitive enteropathy, sprue, regional enteritis, massive jejunal resection, and congenital folate malabsorption, by drug therapy, as with methotrexate, anticonvulsants, and oral contraceptives, and from increased requirements, such as pregnancy, hemolytic anemia, and infancy. The client appears quite ill, thin, and emaciated.

Vitamin B_{12} deficiency is caused by: inadequate diet, as happens with strict vegetarianism or infants of B_{12} deficient mothers; lack of the intrinsic factor, as in pernicious anemia, total or partial gastrectomy, congenitally abnormal intrinsic factor, or diffuse gastric damage; jejunal bacterial overgrowth; or ileal dysfunction, for instance regional enteritis, ileal resection, tropical sprue, ileal tuberculosis (TB), radiation ileitis, and lymphoma of the ileum.

The same basic etiological factors—dietary inadequacies, impaired absorption, and metabolic disturbances—underlie both vitamin B_{12} deficiency and folic acid deficiency.

Laboratory Studies. Diagnosis is made by finding a low RBC count, high number of megaloblasts in the bone marrow, elevated unconjugated bilirubin, and elevated LDH. The Schilling test detects the lack of intrinsic factor and is positive in pernicious anemia.

Medical Interventions. Treatment is to administer oral or parenteral vitamin B_{12} and folic acid until symptoms abate. In addition, the primary cause of the anemia needs to be corrected.

Nursing Interventions. The client needs to be instructed on proper dietary habits. He should eat foods high in iron, protein, and vitamins.

Decreased Red Blood Cell Precursors

Aplastic Anemia

Pathophysiology. Aplastic anemia is a deficiency of circulating erythrocytes because of the arrested development of RBCs within the bone marrow. It results from an injury to the hematopoietic precursor cell, the pluripotent stem cell. Although aplastic anemia sometimes occurs alone, it is usually accompanied by agranulocytosis (a reduction in leukocytes) and thrombocytopenia. These three problems occur together because the bone marrow produces not only RBCs but white blood cells (WBCs) and platelets as well. Consequently, if the bone marrow is abnormal for any reason or if it has suffered exposure to a myelotoxin (any substance that is toxic and damaging to bone marrow), production of erythrocytes, leukocytes, and thrombocytes slows greatly, and a deficiency of all three types of cells develops; this condition is called pancytopenia.

Etiology. The incidence of aplastic anemia is approximately four cases per million population. It can be due to a variety of agents. In approximately one-half of clients, the etiology of aplastic anemia is unknown. Injury to the stem cell, direct injury to the essential hematopoietic microenvironment of the bone marrow, or specific suppression of hematopoiesis by an immunological suppressor mechanisms are just a few known etiologies of aplastic anemia. Specific myelotoxins are radiation, benzene, alkylating agents, antimetabolites, chloromycetin (26 percent of the cases), sulfonamides, anticonvulsants, and insecticides. The mechanism of the damage inflicted by these agents, which unpredictably and sporadically produce severe marrow injury, is unknown. Several possibilities include a metabolic effect on cellular differentiation or an autoimmune mechanism directed against immature hematopoietic precursor cells and activated by the drug.

Clinical Presentations and Nursing Assessments. The onset may be insidious or rapid. In idiopathic cases, the onset is usually gradual. When bone marrow failure is the result of a myelotoxin, however, the onset may be explosive and the client may quickly develop distressing symptoms.

Laboratory Studies. The client will have a normocytic anemia with progressive fatigue, lassitude, and dyspnea. He will have a granulocytopenia and suffer from an increased susceptibility to infection. He will be thrombocytopenic and suffer from a bleeding disorder.

Medical Interventions. The treatment of the disease depends on the severity. Any potentially toxic agent or drug should be discontinued. Clients should have frequent hemograms if being treated therapeutically with myelotoxins. Blood transfusions are the mainstay of therapy. However, transfusions are discontinued as soon as the bone marrow begins to produce RBCs. Transfusion for anemia must be used only when the anemia causes real physiological disability, or when bleeding is life threatening due to platelet deficiency. Unneeded transfusion increases the opportunity for development of immune reactions to platelets, shortens the transfused life span of this formed element, and may increase the rate of rejection to transplanted marrow cells if this course of treatment is subsequently elected. Repeated transfusions can result in hemosiderosis and an enlarged spleen. Extensive trials have been performed with chelating agents. They are used as a substitute method for iron removal in clients whose anemia is severe enough to preclude a phlebotomy. Corticosteroids and androgens are sometimes prescribed on a trial basis to help stimulate bone marrow function. Platelet concentrates may be transfused for life-threatening thrombocytopenia, but the emergence of antiplatelet antibodies may decrease their effectiveness. Careful attention to HLA typing of donor platelets can alleviate the problems of sensitization.

Splenectomy is considered when the client has an enlarged spleen that is either destroying normal RBCs or supressing the development of RBCs within the bone marrow.

Bone marrow transplantation can be performed for those clients who have a matched sibling. Clients who survive bone marrow transplantation for aplastic anemias are capable of living totally normal, healthy lives.

Nursing Interventions. The prevention and treatment of complications resulting from pancytopenia are the most important parts of nursing care. The two major complications are infections and bleeding (see Chaps. 5 and 8).

Myelophthisis

Myelophthisis is a condition where decreased RBC precursors are caused by bone marrow replacement by nonmarrow elements. This occurs in leukemia, tumor cells, infectious granulomas, fibrous tissue replacement, or lipid storage cell replacement. The anemia is normocytic and normochromic. The anemia may be secondary to local competition between invading cells to hematopoietic cells for essential nutrients. The treatment is to eliminate the primary disease.

Decreased Erythropoietic Effect

Anemia of Chronic Disease

Pathophysiology. One situation in which clinical disorders result from a decreased erythropoietin effect is the anemia of chronic disease. It accompanies such diseases as chronic infections, especially TB, connective tissue disorders, malignancy, extensive trauma, or surgery. It can also accompany uremia. The life span of the RBC is short. The defect is not in the RBC, but is extracorpuscular.

Clinical Presentations and Course. On the average, clients with the anemia of chronic disease have lower plasma and urinary erythropoietin levels, for the degree of anemia, than do patients with anemia due to other causes. The anemia may be primarily a disorder of iron supply to the erythroid cell. A disturbance in iron metabolism is clearly present. It develops slowly, and may be hard to differentiate from iron deficiency. The anemia is mild, mean corpuscular volume (MCV) is normal, and RBCs are normochromic and normocytic. Reticulocyte count is normal or decreased. Serum levels of iron and total iron binding capacity (TIBC) are depressed. Marrow aspiration shows abundant iron with characteristic morphological abnormality. Because this anemia develops slowly, it is well tolerated by the client and does not require blood transfusions. Nursing care is that for the anemic client (Chap. 13).

Increased Destruction of Red Blood Cells

Increased destruction of RBCs can be intrinsic to the RBC or extrinsic to the RBC. Intrinsic RBC abnormalities include the abnormal Hgbs, defective glycolysis, and membrane abnormalities. Extrinsic causes incude prosthetic heart valves, thrombotic thrombocytopenia purpura, infectious agents, and other causes.

Abnormal Hemoglobin
Abnormal Hgbs represent a large proportion of anemias secondary to increased destruction of RBC. Hgb variants are inherited as an autosomal codominant trait. Abnormal Hgb is usually detected by electrophoresis. They are classified as follows: sickle cell trait; sickle cell anemia; unstable Hgb variants; variants with high oxygen affinity; and Hgb M. Some of these will be discussed.

Sickle Cell Anemia
Sickle cell anemia is a chronic hereditary hemolytic disorder. It is characterized by the presence of Hgb S instead of Hgb A. It can exist in the anemia form and in trait form.

About 8 percent of black Americans are heterozygous for Hgb S. The RBCs contain Hgb S and Hgb A. In the sickle cell trait, the individuals rarely develop crises, and only when severely hypoxic. However, these clients often do display impaired ability to concentrate urine, and occasionally have recurrent episodes of painless hematuria due to renal medullary infarction.

Pathophysiology. In sickle cell anemia, upon deoxygenation, a RBC containing Hgb S acquires an elongated crescent or sickle shape. It becomes rigid and obstructs capillary blood flow, leading to local tissue hypoxia, further deoxygenation of Hgb, and therefore further sickling. This vicious cycle may amplify microscopic obstructions into a large infarction. Ordinarily, sickled cells resume a normal shape upon reoxygenation. However, membranes of sickled red cells may become damaged, with resulting formation of irreversibly sickled cells. Continuous formation and destruction of these cells contributes to the severe hemolytic anemia occurring in sickle cell anemia. Two factors that promote sickling are increased 2, 3 DPG and acidosis. In addition, increased MCHC promotes sickling.

Hypoxia develops in persons with Hgb S whenever they are exposed to low oxygen tensions as a result of climbing to high altitudes, flying in non-pressurized planes, exercising strenuously, or undergoing anesthesia without receiving adequate oxygenation. Although both Hgb S and Hgb A have the same solubility when oxygenated, deoxygenation of the blood drastically affects Hgb S. Thus, when normal Hgb is deoxygenated, it becomes only half as soluble as when oxygenated, whereas Hgb S becomes 50 times less soluble. The decreased solubility of Hgb S causes it to become more viscous and to crystallize, thereby deforming the shape of the cell. The heavy concentration of misshapen cells during a sickling crisis makes the blood abnormally viscous; as a result, the circulation becomes extremely sluggish. If dehydration due to vomiting, diarrhea, excessive sweating, or ingestion of diuretics is also present, the blood becomes even thicker and the pathological situation is compounded.

Symptoms are due to the following three underlying factors: hemolytic anemia resulting from the destruction of sickle cells; thrombosis and infarction owing to occlusion of the microcirculation by the sickled cells; and an elevated bilirubin owing to the release of Hgb. These three problems profoundly affect all the organs and tissues of the body with severe often fatal consequences.

Clinical Presentations. Clinically, the client will have impaired growth and development, failure to thrive, increased tendency to develop serious infections, especially opportunistic infections, marked impairment of splenic function with inadequate clearance of blood-borne bacteria, and severe hemolytic anemia. Morbidity and mortality is due to the recurrent vasoocclusive phenomena, with painful crises and chronic organ damage. The spleen develops recurrent infarcts and becomes fibrotic. The vasoocclusive phenomena can be divided into painful crises and chronic organ damage.

Painful crises may appear suddenly in any part of the body, but are common in the abdomen, chest, and joints. Frequently, the painful crises are preceded by viral or bacterial infection.

Chronic organ damage is due to the cumulative effect of recurrent vasoocclusive episodes. Any organ or system may be involved. In the cardiopulmonary system, impairment of pulmonary function is common. Clients have hypoxemia due, in part, to intrapulmonary arterial–venous shunting. Congestive heart failure develops frequently from the burdens of chronic severe anemia and hypoxemia. In the hepatobiliary system, icterus and increased tendency to form gallstones commonly results from chronic hemolysis. In the genitourinary system, the hypertonic and acidic environment in the renal medulla promotes sickling with resulting microinfarcts. The clients may develop significant and prolonged painless hematuria. In the skeletal system, bone infarcts produce biconcave fish mouth vertebrae, which are characteristic of the disease. Aseptic necrosis of the femoral head is common, and osteomyelitis is frequent, with *Salmonella* a common cause. Ocular complications include retinal infarcts, peripheral vascular disease, and retinal detachment. Skin changes occur in the form of chronic ulcers, particularly in severely anemic clients. In the nervous system, one-quarter of all clients eventually develop some neurological complications. Hemiplegia is the most frequent.

Laboratory Studies. Diagnosis is made from the appearance of the blood smear. Hemoglobin electrophoresis shows the sickled Hgb.

Medical Interventions. Treatment is supportive. Infection is treated with antibiotics and preventative measures. Clients are given folic acid replacement because they have an increased folic acid requirement. Painful crises should be treated promptly with analgesia and hydration. Because crises may be aborted if treated early, it is advisable to give clients a supply of analgesics that can be self-administered. Blood transfusions have a limited role in the management of sickle cell anemia. Between crises, clients usually tolerate anemia well. Genetic counseling may be useful in the prevention of sickle cell anemia. In the United States, an increasing number of patients are surviving into adulthood and bearing offspring.

Nursing Interventions. Nursing care revolves around educating the client that he carries the sickle cell trait and can transmit it to his offsprings. Persons having only the sickle cell trait may never be detected unless they are exposed to extremely low oxygen tensions. However, extremely hard work or exercise, or such stress as pregnancy may cause the trait to be evidenced through collapse or other effects.

Unstable Hemoglobin
Over 60 unstable Hgb variants are known. These Hgbs cause hemolysis in heterozygous subjects. The homozygous state is probably lethal. These variants constitute a large group of amino acid substitutions in Hgb chains, each of which results in an unstable compound that denatures spontaneously or when exposed to oxidant drugs. The amino acid substitutions distort the structure of Hgb. The Hgbs readily autooxidize to methemoglobin whereupon the heme becomes detached and residual relatively insoluble globin forms an intracellular precipitate, or Heinz body. The precipitates distort and make rigid the RBC membrane. The cell then becomes trapped in the reticuloendothelial system. The entire cell is destroyed, or the precipitate is pitted from the RBC. Chronic hemolytic anemia of variable severity, often accelerated by drugs or infection

and displaying Heinz body formation, is typical of these disorders. The abnormal Hgb is usually detected by heat precipitation. Management consists principally of avoiding oxidant drugs.

Defective Glycolysis

Anemias resulting from defective glycolysis are pyruvate kinase deficiency and G6PD deficiency. RBC energy requirements are met by glucose metabolism. There is no Krebs cycle in RBC metabolism. RBC glucose is catabolized either by anaerobic glycolysis, the Embden-Myerhof pathway, to pyruvate and lactate, or by the pentose phosphate pathway (hexose monophosphate shunt), which generates carbon dioxide directly. Functionally abnormal mutants of many of the enzymes of the Embden-Meyerhof and the pentose phosphate pathways are known. Of these, deficient G6PD activity constitutes over 95 percent of the clinically important inherited metabolic defects of the erythrocyte. The next most common RBC enzyme disorder is pyruvate kinase (PK) deficiency.

Glucose-6-Phosphate Dehydrogenase (G6PD) Deficiency

G6PD is an important RBC enzyme. The specific detrimental effect upon erythrocytes is to make them more susceptible to hemolysis following ingestion of those drugs and foods classified as chemical oxidants. An inherited sex linked disorder, G6PD deficiency is a common problem.

Pathophysiology. G6PD deficiency causes hemolysis of RBCs because erythrocytes require glucose for energy; the enzyme G6PD is responsible for about 10 percent of the glucose metabolized by the erythrocytes. When RBCs are exposed to oxidative foods and drugs, the amount of glucose that the RBC must metabolize is greatly increased. If a G6PD deficiency exists, the RBCs are unable to adequately metabolize glucose and consequently, they cannot cope with the oxidative effects of certain substances. As a result, hemolysis occurs. Because young, newly released erythrocytes contain a substantial amount of G6PD, only aging RBCs are destroyed upon exposure to causative agents.

More than 40 oxidative drugs and foods produce hemolytic anemia in persons with G6PD deficiency, e.g., primaquine, quinine, aspirin, sulfonamides, phenacetin, vitamin K derivative, chloramphenicol, thiazide diuretics, and the fava bean.

Clinical Presentations and Nursing Assessments. Following exposure to any of the above agents, the individual with G6PD deficiency develops acute intravascular hemolysis lasting about 7 to 12 days. During this acute phase, the client suffers from anemia and jaundice. Laboratory findings include moderate hemoglobinemia with hemoglobinuria, an elevated serum bilirubin, reticulocytosis, and the appearance of Heinz bodies within the RBC. Following the acute hemolytic stage, the client's blood picture automatically begins to improve, whether or not the offending drug is discontinued. The hemolytic reaction is self-limiting because only older erythrocytes are destroyed.

Medical Interventions. Treatment involves the identification and total removal of the drug or food precipitating the hemolytic reaction.

Nursing Interventions. Care of the client during the week of acute hemolysis is symptomatic, i.e., rest, fluids, and a nutritious diet.

Because drugs that precipitate hemolytic reactions are common and because G6PD has a high worldwide incidence, screening tests should be part of every public health program. It is important that persons be screened for G6PD deficiency before donating blood as administration of cells deficient in G6PD can be hazardous for the recipient.

Pyruvate Kinase Deficiency
Pyruvate kinase deficiency is a rare autosomal recessive deficiency that produces hemolytic anemia only in the homozygous state. Deficiency of the enzyme seriously compromises glycolysis and decreases ATP production. Reticulocytes suffer less severely from this deficiency than do mature erythrocytes. Affected persons manifest anemia and jaundice in childhood. Exchange transfusion may be required. Drugs are not implicated in the pathogenesis. Biliary complications are not uncommon. Moderate splenomegaly is usual, and splenectomy frequently is accompanied by lessening of the transfusion requirement. Precise diagnosis requires enzyme assay. Nursing care is that for the anemic client.

Membrane Abnormalities
The RBC membrane is a dynamic structure, chemically complex, and containing components responsible for a wide variety of functional properties. Accelerated hemolysis due to abnormalities at the RBC membrane may be acquired or hereditary.

Hereditary Spherocytosis
Hereditary spherocytosis is a common form of chronic hemolytic anemia found in all races and all ages. The condition is inherited as a simple mendelian dominant trait.

Pathophysiology. The two most distinct characteristics of hereditary spherocytosis are the appearance of large numbers of spherical shaped erythrocytes and an enlarged spleen. Spherocytosis develops because the erythrocytes have a defective cellular membrane, extremely permeable to the influx of sodium. To curtail the flow of sodium ions through its defective membrane, the erythrocyte must increase its metabolic work and consequently, its expenditure of glucose. Glucose and cellular energy become depleted and sodium ions flow in without meeting resistance. The RBC interior becomes hypertonic, causing the erythrocyte to swell by drawing water to the cell. Because spherocytes are thick and relatively inflexible, they are easily trapped within the spleen where they are devoured by phagocytes. As a result the spleen becomes greatly enlarged from overwork and the client suffers from anemia and jaundice as a result of the massive hemolysis of RBCs within the spleen.

Clinical Presentations and Nursing Assessments. Symptoms are the same as the general symptoms of hemolytic anemia: malaise, anemia, jaundice, gallstones, and splenomegaly. Because of the massive size of the spleen, clients with this disorder experience left upper quadrant pain and fullness.

Laboratory Studies. Laboratory findings include: spherocytes in the blood smear, reticulocytosis, lowered RBC count and Hgb, and increased osmotic fragility. Osmotic fragility is increased because the spherocyte has a smaller surface area than the normal RBC and a larger cell content than normal because of the excessive inflow of water and sodium into the cell. As a result of these two factors, spherocytes rupture quickly when placed in hypotonic saline solutions, because they cannot tolerate a further influx of water.

Medical Interventions. The only treatment indicated in all cases of hereditary spherocytosis is splenectomy. Ninety percent of clients who undergo splenectomy experience complete reversal of symptoms. Although spherocytes continue to circulate, these misshaped cells usually have a more normal life span once the spleen is removed. Nonetheless, this condition cannot be completely cured.

The administration of blood transfusions may benefit the client in hemolytic crises.

Nursing Interventions. Nursing care is directed at conserving the energy of an anemic client.

Other Anemias Due to Membrane Abnormalities
Other RBC membrane disorders are hereditary elliptocytosis and alpha beta lipoproteinemias. Clinical effects vary from mild to severe hemolysis due to membrane defect. Paroxysmal nocturnal hemoglobinuria is another acquired RBC membrane disorder. This disorder is a hemolytic anemia mediated by the complement system. However, it does not involve antibody immune mechanisms. It may be the result of an injury at the level of the pluripotent stem call. Pancytopenia is common, but the diagnostic finding is the presence of populations of RBCs sensitive to the hemolytic action of complement. The diagnosis involves finding a history of anemia and dark urine on awakening (nocturnal hemoglobinuria), hemolysis with iron deficiency, and pancytopenia. There is a high incidence of thromboembolic disease associated with this disorder. Aplastic anemia and acute leukemia may occur. Treatment is supportive and directed at the alleviation of symptoms. Administer RBCs that have

been washed with saline, if necessary. Nursing care for these clients is that for an anemic client.

Anemia Due to Other Causes—Extrinsic to the RBC

Anemia can be due to physical factors, for instance malfunctioning prosthetic heart valves or thrombotic thrombocytopenic purpura, antibody destruction of RBCs for instance in autoimmune hemolytic anemia, infectious agents and toxins, and other causes, for instance hypersplenism or osmotic and physical injury. Some of these situations will be discussed here.

Physical Causes of Anemia. Physical injury to RBCs leads to fragmentation and production of schistocytes, hemolysis, release of free hemoglobin into plasma (intravascular hemolysis), and loss of iron via the urine (hemosiderinuria).

Cardiac valve defects can cause hemolysis by exposing blood to severe turbulence, jets of refluxed blood, and impact against underendothelialized surfaces, both natural and plastic. Sheer stress tears RBCs apart. It is also called macroangiopathic hemolytic anemia.

Hemolysis in the arteriolar circulation (microangiopathic hemolytic anemia) may result from damage to arteriolar endothelium or from fibrin deposition within the vessel. Causes include disseminated intravascular coagulation, localized intravascular coagulation, certain renal vascular disorders, and other forms of vasculitis. Thrombotic thrombocytopenic purpura leads to a hemolytic anemia with fragmented RBCs.

Antibody Destruction of RBC

Pathophysiology. There are a number of conditions that lead to antibody destruction of RBCs. Autoimmune hemolytic anemia and drug-induced autoimmune hemolysis are the most common. The autoimmune hemolytic anemias are a group of hemolytic anemias in which shortened RBC life span is mediated by components of the immune system directed at the client's own RBCs. They are acquired disorders with premature RBC destruction. Diagnosis is based on evidence that the antibody, usually IgG, or one or more components of the complement system, is attached to the client's RBCs. There are two theories to the etiology of these disorders. One is that the pathogenesis occurs in the RBC membrane and the normal immune response is stimulated to react to this new antigen. Another possibility is that the defect occurs in the immune system wherein the ability to recognize self is lost or impaired. Whatever the reason, the RBC is recognized as foreign and destroyed by the immune system.

Clinical Presentations and Nursing Assessments. A significant number of clients are initially diagnosed when they cannot be cross-matched for transfusion. They may become severely anemic when bone marrow function is suppressed by mild infections. Any stressful situation accelerates it. Icterus may be present.

Diagnosis is made by the direct Coombs' test. In this test, the client's RBCs are mixed with Coombs' serum, a rabbit antibody. If particular proteins are attached to the RBCs, Coombs' serum causes visible agglutination. For this reason, immune hemolytic anemias are synonymous with Coombs' positive hemolytic anemia.

There are two types of immune hemolytic anemias, warm and cold. This classification is based on whether the antibody functions at body temperature (warm antibody) or below body temperature (cold antibody).

Laboratory Studies. Warm antibodies are usually IgG. The hemolytic anemia caused by warm antibodies may be found in all age groups, but it has a higher incidence for the older age groups. This is probably because it has a high association with lymphoproliferative disorders. It can also be associated with systemic lupus erythematosus. Twenty percent of cases are drug induced. Most severely affected clients have a strongly reactive Coombs' test. Clinically, the severity of this anemia varies from mild chronic hemolysis readily compensated by marrow erythroid hyperplasia, to fulminating hemolysis with prostration, jaundice, and profound anemia.

Medical Interventions. Treatment of the warm type immune hemolytic anemia depends on the clinical severity. Steroids are the first-line treatment, and are temporarily effective in 80 percent of patients. Splenectomy is considered if steroid therapy fails, and if major splenic sequestration can be demonstrated. If splenectomy fails, or is inappropriate, immunosuppressive therapy may be instituted.

Cold reactive autoantibodies are usually IgM in type. Cold-reactive IgM is a complement-fixing agglutinin. It agglutinates RBCs in the distal vasculature at low ambient temperatures, producing a Raynaud-like reaction. Brisk intravascular hemolysis can occur, but is rare. Hemolysis is usually mild. Affected individuals are often in the older age groups. It occurs in association with certain infectious disorders, particularly *Mycoplasma pneumoniae* and infectious mononucleosis, in assocation with lymphoproliferative disease, and idiopathically.

Treatment is supportive. Antibody titers may be decreased with an alkylating agent. Splenectomy and steroid therapy is not effective. The best therapy is preventative by the avoidance of cold. In clients whose cold agglutinin syndrome is associated with lymphoproliferative disorders, improvement may follow anti-leukemic or anti-lymphoma therapy.

Drug-induced Autoimmune Hemolysis

Drug-induced autoimmune hemolysis occurs in clients on high doses of penicillin. It is frequently due to IgG antipenicillin antibodies that react with penicillin bound to the client's RBCs. Anemia may be mild to severe. There are certain IgM antibodies that act against other drugs, including quinine, quinidine, sulfonamides, and phenacetin. The antibodies react with the drug in the serum, forming antigen–antibody complexes that are then absorbed to RBC membranes. Complement fixation is promoted and hemolysis results.

Ten to twenty percent of clients receiving methyldopa for protracted periods have a positive direct antiglobulin (Coombs') test and hemolytic anemia. The drug itself is not directly responsible for the positive test because the antibody lacks any antidrug activity. Withdrawal of methyldopa leads to a gradual decrease in the stength of the Coombs' reaction, and amelioration of the anemia results.

Other Causes of RBC Destruction

Infectious agents and toxins, particularly malaria, clostridia, and snake venom have been known to cause RBC destruction. Other factors implicated are hypersplenism, osmotic injury, for instance infusions of hypotonic solutions, and physical injury, for instance heat and burn injury.

Polycythemia

Polycythemia is a sustained increase in blood Hgb concentration (to about 18 g per 100 ml or more), red count (to 6 million per cu mm or more), or HCT (to 55 percent or more). There are no specific etiologies; polycythemia occurs in a variety of conditions. Absolute polycythemia is when there is an absolute increase in RBC mass, whereas relative polycythemia refers to conditions in which the Hct, Hgb level, or RBC count is elevated because of a decrease in plasma volume but the RBC mass is normal. Polycythemia vera is a myeloproliferative disease in which increased RBC mass is one of several manifestations of panmyelosis.

Pathophysiology. Polycythemia is not due to prolonged RBC survival but from a sustained increase in the level of erythropoiesis in the bone marrow. Relative polycythemia is associated with water deprivation, fluid and electrolyte abnormalities, plasma loss, and burns. Absolute polycythemia is associated with low arterial oxygen saturation, with decreased oxygen transport by hemoglobin or increased affinity for oxygen by abnormal hemoglobins, failure of tissue perfusion, or decreased tissue oxygen utilization. Recall that the predominant control of erythropoiesis is mediated through alterations in tissue oxygen tension. Hypoxia, specifically in the kidney, is believed to lead to an increase in the activity of erythropoietin. Polycythemia is also associated with inappropriate erythropoietin elaboration, as in renal diseases, cerebellar hemangioblastoma, hepatoma, uterine fibroids, and androgen administration.

Clinical Presentations and Course. Polycythemia vera is believed to be a form of malignancy analogous to leukemia. The three major hallmarks of this condition are the relentless, unrestrained production of massive numbers of erythrocytes, the production of massive numbers of erythrocytes, the production of excessive myelocytes (leukocytes within the bone marrow), and an overproduction of thrombocytes. The overproduction of all three of these cells lines results in an increase in the viscosity of blood, an increase in the total volume of the blood that may be twice or even three times greater than normal, and a severe congestion of all tissues and organs with blood.

Clinical features are due to increased RBC mass and blood volume. These include: headaches, plethora, pruritus, dyspnea, and hemorrhage, increased blood viscosity, paresthesias, circulatory stagnation, thrombosis, and hypermetabolism, night sweats, weight loss, and elevated basal metabolism. Splenomegaly is common.

Treatment consists of phlebotomy, myelosuppressive drugs, or radiation. In hypoxic polycythemia, increasing the oxygen content is therapeutic.

CHAPTER 12
Transfusion Therapy

Transfusion therapy is necessary to restore blood volume, to combat shock, to treat severe chronic anemia by increasing oxygen carrying capacity of blood, and to maintain coagulation properties of blood by supplying clotting factors.

WHOLE BLOOD REPLACEMENT

Use of whole blood is restricted to two situations: neonatal total blood exchange and acute massive blood loss. It has a volume of about 500 cc (Table 12–1).

Whole blood is usually collected in citrate–phosphate–dextrose (CPD) anticoagulant preservative solution. Citrate acts as an anticoagulant by binding ionized calcium, without which blood cannot clot. This blood is suitable for transfusion anytime within a 21-day storage period. The 21-day limit is based on posttransfusion survival of red blood cells (RBC) in the recipient's circulation. During this storage period, some alterations occur in the character of the stored blood and these may lead to complications in clients who are massively transfused. Such complications include coagulation disturbances, hypocalcemia, hyperkalemia, acid–base imbalances, ammonia intoxication, and 2,3-DPG loss.

Coagulation disturbances may occur due to the poor survival of platelets, and factors V and VIII in banked blood. Platelets do not survive beyond 24 hours of storage in whole blood. Factors V and VIII both deteriorate in stored blood. Platelet count in adults transfused with 12 to 14 units of stored blood has been found to decrease to 50,000. This platelet decrease can be caused by dilution and washout of client's blood with platelet poor stored blood, by clumping of platelets in clots at injured and operative sites, by trapping of platelets within intravascular aggregations, or by antiplatelet antibodies in the client's plasma. Fresh whole blood provides all components including platelets and coagulation factors.

TABLE 12-1. BLOOD COMPONENTS

Component	Comments
Whole blood	For massive blood loss, 500 cc
Packed cells	For treatment of severe anemia, 250 cc ↓ chance of circulatory overload
Buffy coat red cells	Plasma and white cell layer removed to ↓ incidence of allergic reactions
Washed red cells	Platelet and leukocyte antigens removed
Fresh frozen plasma	Plasma contains coagulation factors until thawed.
Cryoprecipitate	Factors VIII, XIII, and fibrinogen hemophiliacs, Von Willebrand's Disease
Platelets	For thrombocytopenia, give as rapidly as possible
White blood cells	For leukopenia, controversial

Another potential, though rare, complication of massive transfusion is citrate intoxication. Because the calcium binding property of the citrate in the anticoagulant preservative solution can cause a significant decrease in the ionized calcium level, symptoms such as hyperactive muscle reflexes, carpopedal spasms, tetany, and EKG changes can develop. Although citrate intoxication is rarely encountered, it may occur in massive transfusions of CPD blood if the total blood volume is exchanged too rapidly. Also, because citrate is metabolized in the liver and excreted in the kidneys, intoxication may occur with smaller transfusions in persons with hepatic or renal disease. Hypothermia retards citrate metabolism and therefore may contribute to intoxication. Excessive citrate may bind virtually all available ionic calcium, resulting in hypocalcemia. Treatment for this is to administer calcium gluconate (10 ml of 10 percent calcium gluconate per liter of blood) when the blood is given more rapidly than one unit every 5 minutes. Too vigorous replacement of calcium can cause cardiac dysfunction, particularly ventricular fibrillation.

Potassium levels are increased in banked blood. Potassium concentration in a liter of stored blood gradually increases from 3 to 5 mEq/L to 15 to 20 mEq/L. This is due to a release of potassium into the plasma with RBC lysis. Hyperkalemia is rarely noted unless the client is predisposed to retain potassium. When stored blood is used, both the rate of transfusion and the client's ability to handle excess potassium must be considered. To prevent hyperkalemia in clients at risk, fresh blood or blood less than 7 days old should be used.

Stored blood gradually acidifies. The pH drops from 7 when freshly drawn to 6.6 over 21 days. This may be due in part to a rise in pyruvate and lactate levels. Clients who are massively transfused with banked blood may develop an initial metabolic acidosis, but they often have preexisting acidosis due to decreased tissue perfusion. This is followed gradually by delayed metabolic alkalosis caused by rapid metabolism of citrate and resultant excess bicarbonate ion. It usually corrects itself. Studies have been conducted to determine the effects of the use of sodium bicarbonate intravenously in clients massively transfused with stored blood. In one study, clients were given 44.6 mEq of sodium bicarbonate per 5 units of banked blood. Researchers reported a decrease in mortality among clients who received 20 or more units of blood.

Loss of 2,3-DPG from RBC occurs with blood storage. Normally 2,3-DPG forms a complex with hemoglobin in the deoxygenated state, facilitating oxygen release to the tissues. Decreased 2,3-DPG leads to tighter binding of oxygen to hemoglobin, with a shift of the oxyhemoglobin dissociation curve to the left. Stored blood with low levels of 2,3-DPG may be less efficient in providing oxygen to the tissues and the client may become hypoxic. Although 2,3-DPG regenerates within several hours, a seriously ill client who is massively transfused with stored blood may not attain adequate tissue oxygenation.

Blood ammonia levels also can increase with storage. The increase may be from 50 μg when freshly drawn to 680 μg at the end of 21 days. Clients who are most likely to be affected by the increased ammonia level are those with liver impairment.

Administration of fresh blood is not the only way to prevent these complications but many experts recommend administering one unit of fresh blood for every 4 to 5 units of stored when large amounts of blood must be transfused.

Hypothermia is a potential complication in massive blood transfusions from rapid infusion of large amounts of cold blood. Banked blood usually has a temperature of 6 to 10 degrees Centigrade, which, when transfused, may lead to decreased heart rate, cardiac output, and pH. Warm the blood, but not above 38° C. Once blood is warmed, it must not be refrigerated again.

Circulatory overload is another potential hazard. A person whose potential for increased left ventricular output is impaired by failure may develop a discrepancy between the amount of blood entering and leaving the pulmonary vascular tree when massive amounts of whole blood are transfused.

Of course bacterial or viral infections are always a potential complication with either single or multiple blood transfusions. In massive transfusions, when various donor's blood is involved, client's chance of developing serum hepatitis is increased with each succeeding unit.

PACKED CELLS

Packed cells is the component of choice for clients with severe anemia who do not require restoration of blood volume, for instance for chronic anemia, congestive heart failure, elderly debilitated patients in whom rapid shifts of blood volume are not well tolerated. A unit of packed cells has a volume of 200 to 250 cc. The advantages of packed cell components are: the chance of circulatory overload is diminished; there is a decreased risk of reactions to plasma antigens; less sodium, potassium, ammonium, and citrate is given; the hematocrit is raised higher; and there is possibly a decreased risk of serum hepatitis. The hematocrit of a unit of packed cells varies from 60 to 85 percent whereas that of whole blood is 40 percent. Many specialists think that lower plasma content in packed cells decreases the chance of carrying enough hepatitis virus to be infectious. One unit of packed cells can significantly improve the oxygen carrying capacity of the blood, whereas whole blood cannot due to its volume. When administering packed cells, the line should only be flushed with normal saline. Dextrose in water can cause RBC clumping, swelling, and subsequent hemolysis. Lactated Ringer's leads to clot formation.

"Buffy coat" is the term given to the white cell layer that lies just above the column of red cells when whole blood is centrifuged. For clients who have developed antibodies to leukocyte and platelet antigens and who have febrile transfusion reactions, the plasma and buffy coat can be removed from whole blood. Most nonhemolytic febrile transfusion reactions can be prevented by removing these leukocyte and platelet antigens.

Washed red cells are RBCs with an even lower level of platelet and leukocyte antigens. The procedure to wash RBCs is very expensive, and buffy coat red cells are often just as effective.

FRESH-FROZEN PLASMA

The volume of a unit of fresh-frozen plasma (FFP) is 200 to 250 cc. It consists of plasma that is fresh frozen and can be stored for 12 months. It contains all the coagulation factors. Once thawed, it can be given to replace deficient coagulation factors, or used as volume expansion. Plasma stored without freezing for several days may still contain adequate amounts of factors VII, IX, X, and XI, but not V and VIII. Beyond the hepatitis risk, the major problem with FFP is the large volume of plasma needed to deliver adequate amounts of coagulation factors to severely deficient clients.

CRYOPRECIPITATE

Cryoprecipitate contains factors VIII, XIII, and fibrinogen. It is given to clients deficient in factor VII—hemophiliacs and von Willebrand's disease, for instance. It is prepared from a single donor rather than from plasma pools that carry a high risk of hepatitis virus contamination. Factor VIII is concentrated by freezing a unit of plasma and then thawing it slowly. The resulting cryoprecipitate is collected by centrifugation. Pooled precipitates are further concentrated so that a large amount of factor VIII can be made available in a small volume. Cryoprecipitate from a single donor contains about 75 units of factor VIII activity; lyophilized concentrates containing up to 800 units per vial are diluted in 50 ml of fluid. The initial dose is 1 unit for each 6 kilograms of body weight, followed by half that amount of 6 to 12-hour intervals. The rate of administration is generally 1 unit per 5 minutes. Complications include occasional urticarial reactions, hepatitis, other viral diseases, and vasomotor reactions, for instance febrile reactions with vasoconstriction, chills, and headaches.

Transfusions of factor IX can be given for the treatment of hemophilia B, or Christmas disease. Prothrombin complex, or a solution of factors IX, II, VII, and X, can be given for hemophilia B, severe liver disease, or a deficiency of multiple coagulation proteins. It carries a high risk of hepatitis because it is derived from a large pool of donors.

PLATELET TRANSFUSION

Large amounts of platelets are now readily obtainable from a single donor with the new cell separators available. By using a single donor, the number of antigens to which a recipient is exposed may be reduced; hence, he can receive effective platelet infusions for a longer period of time. Human leukocyte antigen (HLA) matching of donor and recipient also allows more frequent and effective platelet transfusion.

Platelet transfusions are usually given to thrombocytopenic clients with platelet counts of less than 20,000 per cu mm. Clients who are actively bleeding and have platelet counts of less than 50,000 require transfusions also. Other clients who may require platelet transfusion are those whose platelet function has been adversely affected by drugs such as aspirin. Prophylactic platelet transfusions may be given to prevent spontaneous hemorrhage into the brain. Many leukemic clients may have abnormally functioning platelets and serious bleeding may occur with counts of more than 20,000; however, most clients can tolerate counts of 15,000 to 20,000 without hemorrhagic manifestations.

One unit of platelets is derived from 500 ml of whole blood via centrifuge. Platelets survive 8 to 10 days in the recipient's circulation, but the life span of the cell is affected by the clinical situation. The platelet may survive in the leukemic no longer than 1 to 3 days. On the average, one unit of platelets raises the platelet count by 12,000 to 15,000.

The client may not respond to the platelet transfusion due to: immunological barrier to the transfusion; poor platelet preparation; or a factor in the client's clinical status shortening in vivo survival of the platelets, for instance fever, sepsis, disseminated intravascular coagulation (DIC), or splenomegaly. A febrile response to platelet transfusion may be secondary to a reaction of recipient leukoagglutinins with donor-contaminating granulocytes. This leads to antibody formation against leukocytes with allergic symptoms. Platelet concentrates prepared from the blood of random donors without HLA typing predisposes the recipient to an allogenic response. A refractory state occurs when transfusion of viable platelets does not elevate the platelet count due to presence of HLA antigens that stimulate alloimmunization and subsequent platelet cell destruction. The occurrence of a refractory state is inevitable in those who receive multiple transfusions.

As platelet storage time increases, there is a higher incidence of contamination. Transmission of infectious diseases via phlebotomy and cell separator apparatus also creates an increased susceptibility of contracting hepatitis. This is due to the concentrate being derived from multiple donors. The risk of hemolytic reactions also increases in direct correlation with the number of individual donors.

Platelets are administered rapidly, preferably by intravenous (IV) push (bolus). The faster platelets are given, the higher the level of circulating platelets. They are infused like packed cells, with a special filter and Y tubing. Only 3 percent of platelets are lost by passage through these filters. If a standard transfusion set is used for transfusion of multiple platelet packs, the transfusion set should be rinsed with saline to insure that the total dose of platelets is transfused to the patient. Ten units of platelets is approximately 250 cc. The platelet pack should be given as soon as it arrives on the unit—do not refrigerate it.

VOLUME EXPANDERS

Albumin

Plasma albumin constitutes 50 to 60 percent of plasma protein and accounts for most of the oncotic pressure of plasma. It is the chief determinant of plasma volume. Albumin concentrate is available in 5 and 25 percent solutions and is prepared from plasma. They are free from viral contaminants including hepatitis. It is used as a volume expander to expand the blood volume of clients in hypovolemic shock and to elevate the level of circulating albumin in those with hypoalbuminemia. The 25 percent solution should be given slowly (1 ml/min) to prevent rapid expansion of plasma volume with consequent circulatory overload.

Plasmanate and Plasma Protein Fraction

Plasmanate and plasma protein fraction are trade names for solutions of albumin, amino acids, and other materials. They are as useful as albumin for volume replacement and are also hepatitis-free.

Antibody reactions to plasma proteins are too rare to warrant the expense of routine cross-matching. It may occur if the recipient is deficient in IgA and has been sensitized by previous transfusions. The initial reaction may be chills, fever, and hives. Subsequent reactions may be severe. Therefore, the serum IgA levels should be assessed before giving these solutions. Both of these volume expanders are hyperosmolar. They act by pulling fluid into the intravascular space.

WHITE BLOOD CELL TRANSFUSION

White blood cells (WBC) are obtained from normal or leukemic individuals by continuous flow cell separator. The donor is depleted slightly of platelets and not at all of WBCs because the trauma of being on the machine increases the donor's WBC production. The postdonation WBC count is usually higher than the predonation count. The donation takes $3\frac{1}{2}$ hours.

The donor and recipient must be ABO compatible and preferably HLA compatible. HLA compatibility is important with HLA sensitized clients from previous transfusions.

The transfusion will not increase the total WBC count substantially. It will increase the marginal pool of leukocytes, rather than the circulating pool. At the tissue level, WBCs will be more readily available for phagocytosis.

The transfusion is administered slowly, over 2 to 4 hours. The client may have rigors and fever secondary to sensitization to WBC antigens from previous transfusions, or normal bactericidal effects of leukocytes. If an infected person is granulocytopenic, he will not exhibit symptoms of infection until the granulocytes are introduced. Therefore, shaking chills and fever are not serious reactions, and transfusions should not be discontinued because of them. Hives can also occur secondary to allergic responses to plasma proteins. The client can be premedicated with diphenhydramine and hydrocortisone to ameliorate these symptoms. Small doses of meperidine given IV can also be effective. If the client develops hives on the neck, check him frequently for laryngeal edema. This reaction is usually treated with antihistamine (Table 12–2).

TRANSFUSION REACTIONS

Blood transfusions are actually transplantations of tissue from one person to another. It is important that the recipient does not have antibodies to the

TABLE 12-2. MASSIVE TRANSFUSION—COMPLICATIONS

	Clinical Effects
1. Poor survival of platelets and coagulation factors in banked blood	Bleeding
2. Citrate intoxication	↓ Calcium, → hyperactive muscle reflexes, carpopedal spasm, tetany, and ECG changes
3. ↑ Potassium concentration in banked blood	Hyperkalemia
4. ↓ pH in stored blood	Metabolic acidosis
5. ↓ 2,3-DPG in stored blood	Hypoxia
6. ↑ Blood ammonia levels in stored blood	Encephalopathy
7. Cold blood	Hypothermia

donor's RBCs and that the donor does not have antibodies to the recipient's RBCs. If either of these conditions exist, there will be a hypersensitivity reaction, which can vary in severity from mild fever to anaphylaxis with severe intravascular hemolysis. Although typing for the major ABO and Rh antigens does not guarantee that a reaction will not occur, it does greatly reduce the possibility of such a reaction.

There are four types of transfusion reaction: hemolytic, bacterial, allergic, and circulatory overload.

Hemolytic transfusion reactions are usually caused by ABO incompatibility. Rh incompatibility also leads to a hemolytic reaction but this occurs more gradually and may be less severe. Improper storage of blood with wide temperature fluctuations and faulty transfusion procedures, such as the use of dextrose solution, can also cause hemolysis. Experimental evidence suggests that manifestations and sequelae produced by transfusion of incompatible blood are caused by antigen–antibody complexes released into the circulation. Disseminated intravascular coagulation develops with all the expected pathological changes. The entire syndrome can be explained on the basis of triggering of a series of interactions between the coagulation and complement cascades. The antigen–antibody complex activates the classical complement pathway, and the release of histamine and serotonin by mast cells. Platelets may also be involved with the release of histamine and serotonin. Activation of the Hageman factor leads to the formation of bradykinin. The combined action of all of these vasoactive substances has been postulated to mediate the initial hypotension and shock that occurs in the more severe hemolytic transfusion reactions. There is a secondary release of catecholamines that results in vasoconstrictive circulatory reactions. Activation of the Hageman factor results in release of the intrinsic clotting cascade terminating in the conversion of fibrinogen to fibrin by thrombin. Platelets, and perhaps also WBCs and RBC membranes, may contribute by release of thromboplastic substances. Renal damage can thus result from a combination of hypotension and vasoconstriction compromising renal blood flow with deposition of fibrin thrombi. The severity of renal complications is dose dependent. The magnitude of the insult depends on not only the quantity of blood transfused but also on the quality and quantity of antibody present. Renal failure may be mild and transitory with rapid return of urine output, and little alteration in clearance of metabolites to renal failure with acute tubular necrosis, which may not be reversible.

A mild hemolytic transfusion reaction consists of fever and chills and occurs when the offending antibody titer is low, the dose of RBC infused is small, or so large and rapid that antibodies present were swamped and distributed diffusely on the transfused cells. A severe reaction consists of severe back pain, substernal tightness, dyspnea, circulatory collapse, hypotension, urticaria, vomiting, diarrhea, hemoglobinuria, oozing from puncture sites, hemorrhagic diathesis, and renal shutdown.

Allergic reactions are most often seen in clients with a history of allergy. The client may have urticaria, itching, unaccompanied by chill and fever, bronchospasm, or anaphylactoid reactions. It is thought to be related to the presence of atopic substances that are capble of interacting with antibodies present in the donor's or the recipient's plasma.

Febrile reactions occur in clients with antibodies directed against leukocytes. The client usually will have a history of multiple transfusions. The recipient will experience sensations of cold with or without rigors, increased heart rate or temperature, and in severe reactions, hypotension, cyanosis, fibrinolysis, leukopenia, and tachypnea. In the susceptible individual, washed RBCs, or buffy coat poor cells should be given.

Bacterial reactions are seen after transfusion of contaminated blood products. Usually a gram-negative organism is at fault, because these organisms grow rapidly in blood stored at refrigerated temperatures, and release endotoxins. This situation needs to be treated immediately.

Delayed transfusions reactions occur 3 to 21 days after the transfusion. It presents as a mild hemolytic reaction. An offending antibody can be identified in the client's serum.

Treatment of Transfusion Reactions

The most effective treatment of a transfusion reaction is prevention. Extreme caution should be taken with drawing blood for cross-matching, as per hospital policy. Transfusion components should be analyzed for the client's blood type, hospital identification number on the request slip, client armband, and chart. The identification process should be performed by two individuals.

If the client does exhibit signs of a transfusion reaction, the unit of blood should be discontinued and sent back to the blood bank, along with blood and urine samples according to hospital policy. Depending on the severity of the reaction, the recipient may be given mannitol, furosemide, and saline infusions to prevent acute tubular necrosis. A severe transfusion reaction is usually seen only in clients with a history of multiple transfusions. For mild reactions, the client is usually observed closely for signs of impending hemolysis.

CHAPTER 13

Nursing Care of the Anemic Client

The anemic client needs to conserve his energy. This is because the anemic individual has a decreased capacity to carry oxygen in his blood. All nursing measures should be carried out with the preservation of energy in mind.

Goals of care for the client with anemia are to alleviate or control the causative factors, relieve symptoms, prevent complications, and develop, for clients with chronic anemia, a realistic practical lifelong plan of care.

ALTERATIONS IN OXYGENATION: ENERGY DEFICIT DUE TO DECREASED ABILITY TO CARRY OXYGEN

Rest is essential to lower the client's oxygen requirements and to reduce the strain on the heart and the lungs. Clients with mild anemia, although usually asymptomatic, should be encouraged to rest frequently throughout the day, to shorten their work day if possible, and to retire early. If the ambulatory client experiences dizziness or light-headedness while at work, tell him to lie flat for a few minutes. Lying down with a pillow helps to relieve dizziness by increasing the circulation of blood and oxygen to the brain.

Clients with severe anemia are usually hospitalized and placed on bed rest until clinical improvement occurs. An extremely weak client needs help in bathing, turning, eating, and self-care. Also, to ensure sufficient rest, protect the severely anemic client from frequent visitors, continuous telephone interruptions, and excessive noise. Plan frequent rest periods.

POTENTIAL IMPAIRMENT IN SKIN INTEGRITY

Frequent turning is essential for clients with severe anemia if skin breakdown is to be prevented. Because of the reduction in circulating red blood cells, the tissues of the anemic client do not receive adequate amounts of oxygen. Without preventative measures, the resultant tissue hypoxia can quickly lead to decubitus formation.

POTENTIAL ALTERATION IN NUTRITION: LESS THAN BODY REQUIREMENTS

The diet in anemia should be high in protein, iron, and vitamins. These substances are essential for normal erythrocyte formation. Unfortunately, clients with anemia may have little appetite. Anorexia often results from weakness and profound fatigue. Also clients with iron deficiency anemia and other anemias may have difficulty eating because of sore mouth, esophagus, or tongue. Serve frequent small meals. Avoid hot spicy foods. Give oral hygiene before and after meals. Feed the client who is too exhausted to feed himself.

Anemic clients and those who live with them need to be taught how to plan and prepare a nourishing diet at home. To do this, the nurse can arrange for consultation with a dietitian and the client; provide booklets on nutrition and meal planning and discuss these with the client; provide appetizing recipes for foods high in iron, vitamin B_{12}, and other vitamins; or ask the dietitian to help the client to prepare several weeks of sample menus containing nutritious foods.

ALTERATIONS IN ORAL MUCOUS MEMBRANES

Special mouth care is necessary for clients with severe anemia because they often suffer from a sore mouth or tongue. Special oral hygiene measures include cleansing the teeth before and after meals with a soft toothbrush, allowing the client to rinse his mouth with rinses that are cool and slightly alkaline every 2 hours, and lubricating the lips frequently.

POTENTIAL FOR INJURY

Protecting the client from chills and burns is an important nursing function. Because of poor circulation, clients with anemia typically say they feel cold and chilled. Warm clothing and blankets help anemic clients to feel more comfortable. Avoid applying heating pads or hot water bottles because their skin, which is poorly supplied with blood and oxygen, burns easily. Clients may not be aware of any burning sensation.

NURSING CARE PLAN

Nursing Diagnosis: Alterations in oxygenation—Energy deficit due to decreased ability to carry oxygen
Medical Diagnosis: Anemia

Outcome. Signs and symptoms of anemia will be minimized.

Nursing Interventions	Evaluation
1. Allow rest period after nursing activities.	Client will not develop complications of anemia.
2. Assist with bathing, eating, and ambulating.	
3. Counsel visitors about client's need to rest.	
4. Evaluate client every 8 hr for progression or regression in symptoms of anemia.	

Nursing Diagnosis: Potential impairment in skin integrity

Outcome. Clients will express willingness to participate in prevention of the pressure sores.

Nursing Interventions	Evaluation
1. Turn every hour.	Client will not develop decubiti.
2. Encourage client to turn in bed frequently.	
3. Lubricate skin every 4 hr.	
4. Maintain skin in a well cleansed and well hydrated state.	
5. Assess client's skin daily for reddened areas.	
6. Encourage range of motion and frequent ambulation.	

Nursing Diagnosis: Potential alteration in nutrition: Less than body requirements (see Chap. 8)
Nursing Diagnosis: Alterations in oral mucous membranes (see Chap. 8)
Nursing Diagnosis: Potential for injury

Outcome. Client will identify factors that increase potential for injury, and utilize safety measures to prevent injury.

Nursing Interventions	Evaluation
1. Assess for presence of contributing factors—impaired sensation, decreased tactile sensitivity, side effects of medication.	Client will not sustain injury.
2. Teach preventative measures. a. assess temperature of bath water and heating pads prior to use b. use bath thermometers c. assess extremities daily for undetected injuries d. keep feet warm and dry and skin softened with emollient lotion	

Bibliography

Disorders Hemostasis

Barton, J. Nonhemolytic, noninfectious transfusion reactions. *Seminars in Hematology*, 1981, *18*, 95.

Buickus, B. Administering blood components. *American Journal of Nursing*, 1979, *79*, 938–939.

Caplin, M. Disseminated intravascular coagulation: A multisystem problem. *Dimensions of Critical Care Nursing*, 1984, *3*(2), 76–83.

Carlon, G., & Howland, W. (Eds.). *Critical care of the cancer patient*. Chicago: Yearbook Medical, 1985.

Colman, R., Minna, J., & Robboy, S. Disseminated intravascular coagulation: A problem in critical care medicine. *Heart and Lung*, 1974, *3*, 789.

Colman, R., & Hirsh, J. *Hemostasis and thrombosis: Basic principles and clinical practice*. Philadelphia: Lippincott, 1982.

Conrad, M. Diseases transmissible by blood transfusions: Viral hepatitis and other infectious disorders. *Seminars in Hematology*, 1981, *18*, 122.

Cullins, L. Preventing and treating transfusion reactions. *American Journal of Nursing*, 1979, *79*, 935.

Darovic, G. Disseminated intravascular coagulation. *Critical Care Nurse*, 1982, *2*, 36.

Donham, J., & Denning, V. Cold agglutinin syndrome: Nursing management. *Heart and Lung*, 1985, *14*(1), 59–66.

Dressler, D. Understanding and treating hemophilia. *Nursing*, 1980, *80*, 72–74.

Eberhart, R. Progress in thromboresistant materials research. *American Society for Artificial Internal Organs Journal*, 1983, *6*, 45.

Emminizer, S., Klopp, E., & Haver, J. Autotranfusion: Current status. *Heart and Lung*, 1981, *10*, 83.

Greenwalt, T. Pathogenesis and management of hemolytic transfusion reactions. *Seminars in Hematology*, 1981, *18*, 84.

Griffin, J. P. Nursing care of the critically ill cancer patient. In G. Carlon, & W. Howland (Eds). *Critical care of the cancer patient*. Chicago: Yearbook Medical, 1985.

Haubold, A. Blood/Carbon interactions. *American Society for Artificial Internal Organs Journal*, 1983, *6*, 88.

Herring, M., Hubbard, A., Baughman, S., & Smith, D., et al. Endothelium-lined small artery prostheses: A preliminary report. *American Society for Artificial Internal Organs Journal*, 1983, *6*, 93.

Heyman, S. Effects of cardiopulmonary bypass on coagulation. *Dimensions of Critical Care Nursing*, 1985, *4*, 70–80.

Kakkar, V. Efficacy of low-dose heparin prophylaxis. *Current Therapeutic Research*, 1975, *18*, 6.

Kazak, A. Processing blood for transfusion. *American Journal of Nursing*, 1979, 79, 931.

Kelton, J., & Gibbons, S. Autoimmune platelet destruction. Idiopathic thrombocytopenic purpura. *Seminars in Thrombosis and Hemostasis*, 1982, 8, 83.

Jennings, B. Improving your management of DIC. *Nursing*, 1979, May, 79, 60.

Kim, S., Ebert, C., Lin, J., & McRea, J. Nonthrombogenic polymers: Pharmaceutical approaches. *American Society for Artificial Internal Organs Journal*, 1983, *6*, 76.

Lasslo, A., Quintana, R., & Dugdale, M., et al. Development of novel surface-active compounds for prophylaxis against and treatment of thromboembolic complications. *American Society for Artificial Internal Organs Journal*, 1983, *6*, 47.

Leser, D. Synthetic blood: A future alternative. *American Journal of Nursing*, 1982, *82*, 452–456.

Liebhaber, S., & Manno, C. Update on hemoglobinopathies. *Disease a Month*, 1983, July, *29*(10), 1–60.

Long, J., & DeSantis, S. Thrombogenicity and the interaction of proteins, platelets and WBC. *Biomaterials, Medical Devices and Artificial Organs*, 1983, *11*, 63.

Mailar, R., et al. An alternative extrinsic pathway of human blood coagulation. *Blood*, 1982, *60*, 1353.

Mayer, G. Disseminated intravascular coagulation. *American Journal of Nursing*, 1973, 73, 2067.

McGillick, K. DIC: The deadly paradox. *RN*, 1982, Aug., *82*, 41.

Merrill, E., & Salzman, E. Polyethylene oxide as a biomaterial. *American Society for Artificial Internal Organs Journal*, 1983, *6*, 60.

Moake, J., & Funicella, T. Common bleeding problems. *Clinical Symposia*, 1983, *35*, 1.

Munro, M., Eberhart, R., & Maki, N., et al. Thromboresistant alkyl derivatized polyurethanes. *American Society for Artificial Internal Organs Journal*, 1983, *6*, 65.

Neame, P., & Hirsh, J. Increased platelet destruction. *Seminars in Thrombosis and Hemostasis*, 1982, 8, 75.

Parker, A. Massive blood transfusions. *American Journal of Nursing*, 1979, 79, 944.

Rickles, F., & Edwards, R. Activation of blood coagulation in cancer: Trousseau's syndrome revisited. *Blood*, 1983, *62*, 14.

Rooney, A., & Haniley, C. Nursing management of disseminated intravascular coagulation. *Oncology Nursing Forum*, 1985, *12*, 15–22.

Rutman, R., Hyatt, C., Miller, W., & White, E. Screening donors and the phlebotomy procedure. *American Journal of Nursing*, 1979, 79, 926.

Smith, S. Perflourochemicals: Artificial blood. *Dimensions of Critical Care Nursing*, 1984, *3*(4), 198–206.

Storb, R., & Weiden, P. Transfusion problems associated with transplantation. *Seminars in Hematology*, 1981, *18*, 163.

Tabor, P. Antibiotic-related bleeding disorders. *Focus on Critical Care*, 1985, *12*(3), 31–34.

Thomas, S. Transfusing granulocytes. *American Journal of Nursing*, 1979, 79, 942.

Vogelpohl, R. Disseminated intravascular coagulation. *Critical Care Nurse*, 1981, May, *1*, 38.

Wenz, B., & Barland, P. Therapeutic intensive plasmapheresis. *Seminars in Hematology*, 1981, *18*, 147.

Zeluff, G., Natelson, E., & Jackson, D. Thrombocytopenic purpura—Idiopathic and thrombotic. *Heart and Lung*, 1978, *7*, 327.

Nursing Care

Carpenito, L. *Nursing diagnosis: Application to clinical practice.* Philadelphia: Lippincott, 1983.

Fredette, S., & Gloriant, F. Nursing diagnoses in cancer chemotherapy. *American Journal of Nursing*, 1981, *81*, 2013.

Gordon, M. *Nursing diagnosis.* New York: McGraw Hill, 1982.

Kenner, C., Guzzetta, C., & Dossey, B. *Critical care nursing: Body, mind, and spirit.* Boston: Little, Brown, 1981.

Maher, A. A systems approach to nursing the patient with multiple systems failure. *Heart and Lung*, 1981, *10*, 866.

Rogers, M. *Introduction to the theoretical basis of nursing.* Philadelphia: F. A. Davis, 1970.

Sontag, S. *Illness as metaphor.* New York: Farrar, Strauss, Giroux, 1977.

Anatomy and Physiology of Hematopoietic System

Boggs, D., & Winkelstein, A. *White cell manual.* Philadelphia: F. A. Davis, 1975.

Guyton, A. *Textbook medical physiology, (6th ed.).* Philadelphia: Saunders, 1981.

Harker, L. *Hemostasis manual.* Philadelphia: F. A. Davis, 1974.

Hillman, R., & Finch, C. *Red cell manual.* Philadelphia: F. A. Davis, 1974.

Reich, C. *Cellular elements of the blood.* New Jersey, CIBA Pharmaceutical, 1962.

Roitt, I. *Essential immunology.* Boston: Blackwell Scientific, 1980.

Williams, W., Beutler, E., Ersley, A., & Lichtman, M. *Hematology.* New York: McGraw-Hill, 1983.

Disorders of Erythrocytes

Lynch, E., & Jackson, D. Anemia and malignancies. *Heart and Lung*, 1983, *12*, 44.

Luckmann, J., & Sorenson, K. *Medical-surgical nursing.* Philadelphia: Saunders, 1980.

Disorders of Immunity

Abboud, F. Relaxation, autonomic control, and hypertension. *New England Journal of Medicine*, 1976, *294*, 107–109.

Ader, R. A historical account of conditioned immunobiologic responses. In R. Ader (Ed.), *Psychoneuroimmunology.* New York: Academic Press, 1981.

Ader, R., & Cohen, N. Behaviorally conditioned immunosuppression and murine systemic lupus erythematosus. *Science*, 1982, *215*, 1534–1536.

Ader, R., & Cohen, N. Behaviorally conditioned immunosuppression. *Psychosomatic Medicine*, 1975, *37*, 333–340.

Ader, R., Cohen, N., & Bovbjerg, D. Conditioned suppression of humoral immunity in the rat. *Journal of Comparative and Physiological Psychology*, 1982, *96*, 517–521.

Ader, R., Cohen, N., & Grota, L. Adrenal involvement in conditioned immunosuppression. *International Journal of Immunopharmacology*, 1979, *1*, 141–145.

Allen, J., & Mellin, G. The new epidemic—Immune deficiency, opportunistic infections, and Kaposi's sarcoma. *American Journal of Nursing*, 1982, *82*, 1718.

Amery, W. Levamisole. *Lancet*, 1979, *2*, 528.

Anderson, M., Aker, S., & Hickman, R. O. The double lumen Hickman catheter. *American Journal of Nursing*, 1982, *82*, 272–273.

Bach, F., & van Rood, J. The major histocompatibility complex—Genetics and biology. *New England Journal of Medicine*, 1976, *295*, 806.

Ballucci, B. Selected concepts of cancer as a disease: From 1900 to oncogenes. *Oncology Nursing Forum*, 1985, *12*, 69.

Barbach, A., Higby, D., Brass, C., et al. High dose cytoreductive therapy with autologous bone marrow transplantation in advanced malignancies. *Cancer Treatment Reports*, 1983, *67*, 143.

Beisel, W. R., Chairman. Proceedings of a workshop: Impact of infection on nutritional status of the host. *American Journal of Clinical Nutrition*, 1977, *30*, 1203.

Beisel, W. R., & Wannamacher, J. R. Gluconeogenesis, ureagenesis, and ketogenesis during sepsis. *Journal of Parenteral and Enteral Nutrition*, 1980, *4*, 277.

Bellanti, J. Immunology III, Philadelphia: Saunders, 1984.

Bersani, G., & Carl, W. Oral care for cancer patients. *American Journal of Nursing*, 1983, *83*, 533.

Besedovsky, H., DelRey, A., & Sorkin, E. Immunoregulation mediated by the sympathetic nervous system. *Cellular Immunology*, 1979, *48*, 346–355.

Beveridge, T. Cyclosporin A. *Transplantation Proceedings*, 1983, *15*, 433.

Bingham, C. The cell cycle and cancer chemotherapy. *American Journal of Nursing*, 1978, *78*, 1201.

Bird, A. G., & Britton, S. Relationship between Epstein Barr virus and lymphoma. *Seminars in Hematology*, 1982, *19*, 285.

Bistrian, B. R. Interaction of nutrition and infection in the hospital patient. *American Journal of Clinical Nutrition*, 1979, *30*, 1228.

Blackburn, G. L., & Bistrian, B. R. Nutritional care of the injured and/or septic patient. *Surgical Clinics North America*, 1976, *56*, 1195.

Blackburn, G. L., Bistrian, B. R., Maini, B. S., et al. Nutritional and metabolic assessment of the hospital patient. *Journal of Parenteral and Enteral Nutrition*, 1977, *1*, 11.

Blanchard, E., & Young, L. Clinical applications of biofeedback training: A review of evidence. *Archives of General Psychiatry*, 1974, *30*, 573–589.

Borkowsky, W., & Lawrence, H. Effects of human leukocyte dialysates containing transfer factor in the direct leukocyte migration inhibition assay. *Journal of Immunology*, 1979, *123*, 1741.

Bortin, M. M., & Rimm, A. A. for the Advisory Committee of the International Bone Marrow Transplant Registry. Severe combined immunodeficiency disease. Characterization of the disease and results of transplantation. *Journal of the American Medical Association*, 1977, *238*, 591.

Boss, B., Langman, R., Trowbridge, R., & Dulbecco, R. *Monoclonal antibodies and cancer*. New York: Academic, 1983.

Bovbjerg, D., Ader, R., & Cohen, N. Behaviorally conditioned suppressed of a graft-versus-host response. *Proceedings of the National Academy of Sceince*, 1982, 79, 583–585.

Bovbjerg, D., Cohen, N., & Ader, R. Conditioned suppression of a cellular immune response. *Psychosomatic Medicine*, 1980, 42, 73.

Brown, R. E. Interaction of nutrition and infection in clinical practice. *Pediatric Clinics of North America*, 1977, 24, 241.

Burke, B., & Goode, R. Pneumocystis carinii infection. *Medicine*, 1973, 52, 23.

Cahan, M., & Lydhane, N. Bone marrow transplantation at UCLA. *Cancer Nursing*, 1978, Feb., 2, 47.

Camitta, B. M., & Thomas, E. D. (For the International Aplastic Anemia Study Group.). Severe aplastic anemia: A prospective study of the effect of androgens or transplantation on haematological recovery and survival. *Clinical Hematology*, 1978, 7, 537–595.

Carlson, A. Infection prophylaxis in the patient with cancer. *Oncology Nursing Forum*, 1985, 12, 56.

Carpentier, N., Frere, D., Schuh, D., et al. Circulating immune complexes and the prognosis of acute myeloid leukemia. *New England Journal of Medicine*, 1982, 307, 1174.

Cervantes, F., & Rogman, C. Multivariate analysis of prognostic factors in CML. *Blood*, 1982, 60, 1298.

Chandra, R. K., & Newberne, P.M. *Nutrition, immunity and infection: mechanisms of interactions*. New York: Plenum, 1977.

Clift, R. A., Buckner, C. D., Thomas, E. D., & Stork, D. Allogeneic marrow transplantation using fractionated total body irradiation in patients with acute lymphoblastic leukemia in relapse. *Leukemia Research*, 1982, 6, 401–407.

Clowes, G. H. A., (Ed.). Response to infection and injury—Parts I and II. *Surgical Clinics of North America*, 1976, 56, 802.

Cohen, N., Ader, R., Green, N., & Bovbjerg, D. Conditioned suppression of a thymus independent antibody response. *Psychosomatic Medicine*, 1979, 41, 487–491.

Conry, K. Anergy: The hidden danger. *Heart and Lung*, 1982, 11, 85.

Constantian, M. Association of sepsis with an immunosuppressive polypeptide in the serum of burned patients, *Annals of Surgery* 1978, 188, 209.

Constantian, M., Memzoian, J., Nimberg, R., et al. Association of a circulating immunosuppressive polypeptide with operative and accidental trauma. *Annals of Surgery*, 1977, 185, 73.

Cosimi, A. B. The clinical usefulness of antilymphocyte antibodies. *Transplanation Proceedings*, 1983, 15, 583.

Coyle, N. Analgesics at the bedside. *American Journal of Nursing*, 1979, 79, 1554.

Croce, C., & Klein, G. Chromosome translocations and the human cancer. *Scientific American*, 1985, March, 252, 54.

Croft, C. BCG administration and nursing implications. *American Journal of Nursing*, 1979, 79, 315.

Daeffler, R. Oral hygiene measures for patients with cancer. Part III. *Cancer Nursing*, 1981, Feb., 2, 29.

DeVita, V., Hellman, S., & Rosenberg, S. *AIDS*. Philadelphia: Lippincott, 1985.

DeVita, V., Hellman, S., & Rosenberg, S. *Cancer: Principles and practices of oncology*. Philadelphia: Lippincott, 1983.

Dharan, M. Immunoglobulin abnormalities. *American Journal of Nursing,* 1976, *76,* 1626.

Dodd, M. Theoretical basis of immunotherapy. *American Journal of Nursing,* 1979, *79,* 310.

Donley, D. Nursing the patient who is immunosuppressed. *American Journal of Nursing,* 1976, *76,* 1619.

Durack, D. Opportunistic infections and Kaposi's sarcoma in homosexual men. *New England Journal of Medicine,* 1981, *305,* 1465.

Elliott, C. Radiation therapy: How you can help. *Nursing,* 1976, Sept., *76,* 34.

Engel, B. Clinical biofeedback: A behavioral analysis. *Neuroscience and Biobehavioral Reviews,* 1981, *5,* 397–400.

Ersek, M. The adult leukemia patient in the intensive care unit. *Heart and Lung,* 1984, *13,* 183.

Fox, L. Granulocytopenia in the adult cancer patient. *Cancer Nursing,* 1981, *4,* 459–465.

Fritz, G. Biofeedback and attention training to decrease the frequency and intensity of severe hemophiliac hemorrhagic episodes and related pain. *Biofeedback and Self-Regulation,* 1982, *7* (Abstract).

Fruth, R. Anaphylaxis and drug reactions: Guidelines for detection and care. *Heart and Lung,* 1980, *9,* 662.

Gaarder, K., & Montgomery, P. *Clinical biofeedback: A procedural manual for behavioral medicine.* Baltimore: Williams & Wilkins, 1981.

Gale, R. P. Clinical trials of bone marrow transplantation in leukemia. In R. P. Gale, & C. F. Fox (Eds.), *Biology of bone marrow transplantation.* New York: Academic Press, 1980.

Gale, R. P., and the UCLA Bone Marrow Transplant Unit. Current status of bone marrow transplantation in acute leukemia. *Transplant Proceedings,* 1979, *11,* 1920.

Garner, J., & Simmons, B. CDC guidelines for the prevention and control of nosocomial infections. *American Journal of Infection Control,* 1984, *12,* 103.

Gillis, S. Interleukin biochemistry and biology. *Federation Proceedings,* 1983, *42,* 2635.

Goldman, J. New approaches in chronic granulocytic leukemia—Origin, prognosis, and treatment. *Seminars in Hematology,* 1982, *19,* 241.

Gottlieb, M., Schroff, R., Scitanker, H., et al. Pneumocystis carinii pneumonia and mucosal candidiasis in previously healthy homosexual men. *New England Journal of Medicine,* 1981, *305,* 1425.

Gralnick, H. Classification of acute leukemia. *Annals of Internal Medicine,* 1977, *87,* 740.

Greene, W. A. The psychosocial setting of the development of leukemia and lymphoma. *Annals of the New York Academy of Science,* 1966, *125,* 794.

Griffin, J. Nursing care of the critically ill cancer patient. In G. Carlon (Ed.), *The critically ill cancer patient.* Chicago: Yearbook Medical, 1984.

Griffin, J. Acquired immune deficiency syndrome: A new epidemic. *Critical Care Nurse,* 1983, March, *2,* 21.

Groenwald, S. Physiology of the immune system. *Heart and Lung,* 1980, *9,* 645.

Gupta, S., & Good, S. What is immune regulation. *Triangle,* 1981, *20,* 55.

Hershko, C., & Gale, R. P. Graft-versus-host disease scoring system for predicting survival and specific mortality in bone marrow transplantation recipients. In R. P. Gale, & C. F. Fox (Eds.), *Biology of bone marrow transplantation.* New York: Academic, 1980.

Hiebert, J., McGough, M., Rodeheaver, G., et al. The influence of catabolism on immunocompetence in burned patients. *Surgery*, 1979, *86*, 242.

Howard, R. Effect of burn injury, mechanical trauma, and operation on immune defenses. *Surgical Clinics of North America*, 1979, *59*, 199.

Hutchison, M. M. Administration of fat emulsions. *American Journal of Nursing*, 1982, *82*, 275–77.

Ivey, M. F. The status of parenteral nutrition. *Nursing Clinics of North America*, 1979, *14*, 285.

Johnson, W., Ulrich, F., Meguid, M., et al. Role of delayed hypersensitivity in predicting postoperative morbidity and mortality. *American Journal of Surgery*, 1979, *137*, 536.

Johnstone, J. Infrequent infection associated with Hickman catheters. *Cancer Nursing*, 1982, *5*, 125–29.

Keithley, J. Infection and the malnourished patient. *Heart and Lung*, 1983, *12*, 23.

Klemm, P. Cyclosporin A: Use in preventing graft versus host disease. *Oncology Nursing Forum*, 1985, *12*, 25.

Lachman, L. Human interleukin 1: Purification and properties. *Federation Proceedings*, 1983, *42*, 2639.

Lancaster, L. Kidney transplant rejection: Pathophysiology, recognition, and treatment. *Critical Care Nurse*, 1982, Sept., *2*, 50.

Larson, E. *Clinical microbiology and infection control.* Boston: Blackwell Scientific, 1984.

Law, D. K., Dudrick, S. J., & Abdou, N. I. Immunocompetence of patients with protein–calorie malnutrition. *Annals of Internal Medicine*, 1973, *79*, 545.

Lawler, S. Significance of chromosome abnormalities in leukemia. *Seminars in Hematology*, 1982, *19*, 257.

Lawrence, H. Transfer factor. *Advances in Immunology*, 1969, *11*, 195.

Layton, P. B., Gallucci, B. B., & Aker, S. N. Nutritional assessment of allogeneic bone marrow recipients. *Cancer Nursing*, 1981, *4*:127–135.

Levy, R., & Miller, R. Tumor therapy with monoclonal antibodies. *Federation Proceedings*, 1983, *42*, 2650.

Lind, M. The immunologic assessment: A nursing focus. *Heart and Lung*, 1980, 9, 658.

Lister, T., & Robatiner, A. Treatment of acute myelogenous leukemia in adults. *Seminars in Hematology*, 1982, *19*, 172.

Livingston, B. Cancer chemotherapy research. *American Journal of Nursing*, 1967, *67*, 12.

Locke, S. Influence of stress and emotions in human immune response. *Biofeedback and self-regulation*, 1977, *2*, 320 (Abstract).

Lovejoy, N. Biofeedback: A growing role in holistic health. In P. Chinn (Ed.), *Advances in nursing science—Holistic health* (Vol. 2). Germantown: Aspen Systems, 1980.

MacFarlane, D., & Bacon, P. Side effects of drugs: Levamisole-induced vasculitis due to circulating immune complexes. *British Medical Journal*, 1978, *1*, 407.

Mackey, C., & Hopeful, A. Keeping infections down when risks go up. *Nursing*, 1980, June, *80*, 69.

MacLean, L. Host resistance in surgical patients. *Journal of Trauma*, 1979, *19*, 297.

MacLean, L., Meakins, J., Taguchi, K., et al. Host resistance in sepsis and trauma. *Annals of Surgery*, 1975, *182*, 207.

Marino, L. Cancer patients: Your special role. *Nursing*, 1976, Sept., *76*, 26.

Marx, J. Human T cell leukemia virus linked to AIDS. *Science*, 1983, *220*, 806.

Matthay, R., & Greene, W. Pulmonary infections with immunocompromised patient. *Medical Clinics of North America*. 1980, *64*, 529.

Mattia, M., & Blake, S. Hospital hazards: Cancer drugs. *American Journal of Nursing*, 1983, *83*, 758.

Maxwell, M. Scalp tourniquets for chemotherapy induced alopecia. *American Journal of Nursing*, 1980, *80*, 900.

McAdams, C. Interferon, the penicillin of the future? *American Journal of Nursing*, 1980, *80*, 714.

McCaffery, M., & Hart, L. Undertreatment of acute pain with narcotics. *American Journal of Nursing*, 1976, *76*, 1586.

McLeod, B. Immunologic factors in reactions to blood transfusions. *Heart and Lung*, 1980, *9*, 675.

McLoughlin, G., Wu, A., Saproschetz, I., et al. Correlation between anergy and a circulating immunosuppressive factor following major surgical trauma. *Annals of Surgery*, 1979, *190*, 297.

McMullen, K. When the patient is on bleomycin therapy. *American Journal of Nursing*, 1975, *75*, 964.

Meakins, J., Christou, N., Shizgal, H., & MacLean, L. Therapeutic approaches to anergy in surgical patients: Surgery and levamisole. *Annals of Surgery*, 1979, *19*, 286.

Meakins, J., McLean, A., Kelly, R., et al. Delayed hypersensitivity and neutrophil chemotaxis: effect of trauma. *Journal Trauma*, 1978, *18*, 240.

Meakins, J., Pietsch, J., Bubenick, O., et al. Delayed hypersensitivity: Indicator of acquired failure of host defenses in sepsis and trauma. *Annals of Surgery*, 1977, *186*, 241.

Meyers, J. D., & Thomas, E. D. Infection complicating bone marrow transplantation. In L. S. Young, & R. H. Rubin (Eds.), *Clinical Approach to Infection in the Immunocompromised Host*, New York: Plenum, 1981, 507.

Meyers, J. D., McGuffin, R. W., Neiman, P. E., et al. Toxicity and efficacy of human leukocyte interferon for treatment of cytomegalovirus pneumonia after marrow transplantation. *Journal of Infectious Disease*, 1980, *141*, 555–562.

Morrin, B. Cancer Immunology. *Heart and Lung*, 1980, *9*, 686.

Munster, A., Loadholdt, C., & Leary, A. The effect of antibiotics on cell-mediated immunity. *Surgery*, 1977, *81*, 692.

Neiman, P. E., Meyers, J. D., Medeiros, E., et al. Interstitial pneumonia following marrow transplantation for leukemia and aplastic anemia. In R. P. Gale, & C. F. Fox (Eds.), *Biology of Bone Marrow Transplantation*. New York: Academic Press, 1980.

Newlin, N., & Wellisch, D. The oncology Nurse: Life on an emotional roller coaster. *Cancer Nursing*, 1978, *1*, 447.

Nirenberg, A. High dose methotrexate for the patient with osteogenic sarcoma. *American Journal of Nursing*. 1976, *76*, 1776.

Nuscher, R., Baetzer, L., & Rupinec, D. Bone marrow transplantation. *American Journal of Nursing*, 1984, *84*, 764.

Oncology Nursing Society. *Cancer chemotherapy: Guidelines and recommendations for nursing education and practice*. Pittsburgh: 1984.

Pagana, K. The intrigue and challenge of Goodpasture's syndrome. *Heart and Lung*, 1980, *9*, 699.

Patterson, P. Granulocyte transfusion: Nursing considerations. *Cancer Nursing*, 1980, *3*, 101–103.

Pietsch, J., & Meakins, J. Predicting infection in surgical patients. *Surgical Clinics of North Am*, 1979, *59*, 185.

Pietsch, J., Meakins, J., & MacLean, L. The delayed hypersensitivity response: Application in clinical surgery. *Surgery*, 1977, *82*, 349.

Pinkel, D. Treatment of acute nonlymphocytic leukemia. *Cancer*, 1979, *43*, 1128–1137.

Podjasek, J. Respiratory infection in the mechanically ventilated patient—An overview. *Heart and Lung*, 1983, *12*, 5.

Powles, R. L., Clink, H. M., Bandini, G., et al. The place of bone-marrow transplantation in acute myelogenous leukemia. *Lancet*, 1980, *1*, 1047–1050.

Rana, A., & Luskin, A. Immunosuppression, autoimmunity, and hypersensitivity. *Heart and Lung*, 1980, *9*, 651.

Reaman, G. H., Ladisch, S., Echelberger, C., et al. Improved treatment results in the management of single and multiple relapses of acute lymphoblastic leukemia. *Cancer*, 1980, *45*, 3090–3093.

Reich, S. Lung toxicity of anticancer drugs. *Cancer Nursing*, 1981, Feb., *3*, 59.

Rhoads, C., Adcock, M., & Jovanovich, J. Prevention of nosocomial infection in critical care units. *Nursing Clinics of North America*, 1980, *15*, 803.

Rogers, M., Reich, P., Strom, T., & Carpenter, C. Behaviorally conditioned immunosuppression: Replication of a recent study. *Psychosomatic Medicine*, 1976, *38*, 447–51.

Rutman, R., & Miller, W. *Transfusion therapy*. Rorkville, Md.: Aspen, 1985.

Sanders, J. E., Hickman, R. O., Aker, S., et al. Experience with double lumen right atrial catheters. *Journal of Parenteral Enteral Nutrition*, 1982, *6*, 95–99.

Santos, G., & Tutschke, P. J. Prevention and treatment of graft-versus-host disease in man. In R. P. Gale, & C. F. Fox, (Eds.), *Biology of bone marrow transplantation*. New York: Academic Press, 1980.

Santos, G., Elfenhern, G., Tutschke, P. Bone marrow transplantation—Present status. Parts I & II. *Transplantation Proceedings*, 1979, *11*, 182.

Schwitter, G., & Beach, J. Bone marrow transplantation in children. *Nursing Clinics of North America*, 1976, *11*, 49–57.

Shahinpour, N. The patient with systemic lupus erythematosus: Prototype of autoimmunity. *Heart and Lung*, 1980, *9*, 682.

Shizgal, H., Spanier, A., & Kurtz, R. Effect of parenteral nutrition on body composition in the critically ill patient. *American Journal of Surgery*, 1976, *131*, 156.

Shulman, H. M., McDonald, G. B., Matthews, D., et al. An analysis of hepatic venooclusive disease and centrilobular hepatic degeneration following bone marrow transplantation. *Gastroenterology*, 1980, *79*, 1178–1191.

Slade, M., Simmons, R., Yunis, E., & Greenburg, L. Immunodepression after major surgery in normal patients. *Surgery*, 1975, *78*, 363.

Snow, R., et al. Respiratory failure in cancer patients. *Journal of American Medical Association*, 1979, *241*, 2039.

Solomon, G., & Amkraut, A. Psychoneuroendocrinological effects on the immune response. *Annual Review of Microbiology*, 1981, *35*, 155–184.

Solomon, G. F., & Moos, R. H. Emotions, immunity and disease. *Archives of General Psychiatry*, 1964, *11*, 657.

Sophie, L. Meeting the immunologic challenge of transplant nursing. *Heart & Lung*, 1980, *9*, 690.

Stream, P., Harrington, E., Clark, M. Bone marrow transplantation: An option for children with acute leukemia, *Cancer Nursing*, 1980, *3*, 195–199.

Sullivan, K. M., Shulman, H. M., Storb, R., et al. Chronic graft-versus-host disease in 52 patients: Adverse natural course and successful treatment with combination immunosuppression. *Blood*, 1981, *57*, 267–76.

Theofilopoulos, A., & Dixon, F. Immunologic assessment in clinical medicine. *Triangle*, 1981, *20*, 71.

Thomas, E. D., Storb, R., Cleft, R., et al. Bone marrow transplantation. *New England Journal of Medicine*, 1975, *292*, 832–895.

Valentine, A. Caring for the young adult with cancer. *Cancer Nursing*, 1978, Oct., *1*, 385.

Weiden, P. L., & the Seattle Marrow Transplant Team. Graft-vs-host disease in allogenic marrow transplantation. In R. P. Gale, & C. F. Fox (Eds.), *Biology of bone marrow transplantation*. New York: Academic, 1980.

Weiss, R., & Muggia, F. Cytotoxic drug-induced pulmonary disease: Update 1980. *American Journal of Medicine*, 1980, *68*, 259.

Welch, D. Thrombocytopenia in the adult patient with acute leukemia. *Cancer Nursing*, 1978, Dec., 463.

Wellisch, D., & Yager, J. Is there a cancer prone personality? *A Cancer Journal for Clinicians*, 1983, *33*, 145.

Williamson, K. Cisplatin: Delivering a safe infusion. *American Journal of Nursing*, 1981, *81*, 320.

Winston, D. Interstitial pneumonia and cytomegalovirus infections after bone marrow transplantation. In R. P. Gale, & C. F. Fox (Eds.), *Biology of bone marrow transplantation*. New York: Academic, 1980.

Woods, M., Kowalski, J. (Eds.). Symposium on oncologic nursing practice. *Nursing Clinics of North America*, 1982, *17*, 539.

Worthington, B. Effect of nutritional status on immune phenomena. *Journal of the American Dietetic Association*, 1974, *65*, 123.

Wroblewski, S., & Wroblewski, S. Caring for the patient with chemotherapy induced thrombocytopenia. *American Journal of Nursing*, 1981, *81*, 746.

Yasko, J. *Guidelines for cancer care: Symptom management*. Reston, Va.: Reston, 1983.

Index